PIP Joint Fracture Dislocations

Julie E. Adams
Editor

PIP Joint Fracture Dislocations

A Clinical Casebook

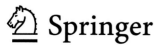 Springer

Editor
Julie E. Adams
Mayo Clinic
Austin, MN, USA

ISBN 978-3-319-28577-1   ISBN 978-3-319-28579-5   (eBook)
DOI 10.1007/978-3-319-28579-5

Library of Congress Control Number: 2016935288

Printed on acid-free paper

This Springer imprint is published by Springer Nature
The registered company is Springer International Publishing AG Switzerland

Preface

Proximal interphalangeal (PIP) joint injuries are common and often unrecognized or unappreciated by the patient or physician. It is important to be able to distinguish between stable, unstable, and tenuous lesions and to understand and appreciate the various options and principles of treatment.

This clinical casebook is a practical handbook that addresses PIP joint injuries and explores principles of treatment. Some of the more common clinical scenarios that may be encountered are described. The book provides a framework for the practicing hand therapist, physician, or surgeon to understand these injuries and choose between treatment options and therapy regimens in order to lead to optimal outcomes. Attention to a stepwise surgical and rehabilitation program is provided.

Chapter topics were chosen to cover the most common and useful areas of pathology and treatment that the surgeon, physician, or therapist may encounter. Chapters are framed in terms of practical principles and case examples to enhance understanding and provide useful guidance to the clinician. Each chapter is designed to highlight clinical pearls and pitfalls and to help the clinician avoid complications and improve outcomes. Expert authors were hand-selected by the editor; these experts were specifically chosen for their expertise and experience in surgery and rehabilitation and their ability to write clear and concise value-packed chapters.

It is my hope that *PIP Fracture Dislocations: A Clinical Casebook* becomes a frequently referenced guide for practicing clinicians and residents, fellows, or students who are interested in a practical appreciation of the issues associated with PIP joint injuries. To that end, I would like to thank the expert authors who have generously contributed to this volume and shared their experience and expertise and who have made my job as editor easy and fun and the fantastic work of Patrick Carr (Springer Developmental Editor) and Kristopher Spring (Springer Publishing Editor) in keeping the work on track and bringing it to fruition. I would also like to thank my husband Scott and our daughter Sarah for their patience and unwavering support.

Austin, MN, USA   Julie E. Adams, M.D.

Contents

Contributors

Julie E. Adams, MD Mayo Clinic, Austin, MN, USA

H.L. Baltzer, MD, FRCS(C) Division of Plastic and Reconstructive Surgery, University of Toronto, Toronto, ON, Canada

O. Alton Barron, MD Department of Orthopedics, CV Starr Hand Surgery Center, Mt. Sinai—Roosevelt Hospital, Mt. Sinai Icahn School of Medicine, New York, NY, USA

Ryan P. Calfee, MD, MSc Department of Orthopedic Surgery, Washington University School of Medicine, St. Louis, MO, USA

Agnes Z. Dardas, BA Department of Orthopedic Surgery, Washington University School of Medicine, St. Louis, MO, USA

Daniel S. Donovan, MD Department of Orthopaedic Surgery, Mt. Sinai-St. Luke's Roosevelt, New York, NY, USA

Reid W. Draeger, MD Department of Orthopaedics, University of North Carolina, Chapel Hill, NC, USA

C. Liam Dwyer, MD Department of Orthopaedic Surgery, UPMC Hamot, Erie, PA, USA

Alex J. Ferikes, MD Department of Orthopaedic Surgery, UPMC Hamot, Erie, PA, USA

Felicity G. Fishman, MD Yale Orthopaedics and Rehabilitation, New Haven, CT, USA

Katie Froehlich, OTR/L, CHT Hand and Upper Body Rehabilitation Center, Erie, PA, USA

Michael P. Gaspar, MD The Philadelphia Hand Center, P.C., Thomas Jefferson University, Department of Orthopaedic Surgery, Philadelphia, PA, USA

Erica J. Gauger, MD University of Minnesota Medical Center, Minneapolis, MN, USA

Sidney M. Jacoby, MD The Philadelphia Hand Center, P.C., Thomas Jefferson University, Department of Orthopaedic Surgery, King of Prussia, PA, USA

Elspeth Kinnucan, MD Department of Orthopaedic Surgery, Kaiser Permanente, Roseville, Roseville, CA, USA

John R. Lien, MD Department of Orthopaedic Surgery, University of Michigan Health Systems, Ann Arbor, MI, USA

Chris Lincoski, MD Department of Orthopedic Hand Surgery, University Orthopedic Center, State College, PA, USA

John D. Lubahn, MD Department of Orthopaedic Surgery, UPMC Hamot, Erie, PA, USA

Steven L. Moran, MD Department of Plastic Surgery, Mayo Clinic Hospital, Rochester, MN, USA

Department of Orthopedic Surgery, Mayo Clinic Hospital, Rochester, MN, USA

Maureen O'Shaughnessy, MD Department of Orthopedic Surgery, Mayo Clinic, Rochester, MN, USA

Marco Rizzo, MD Department of Orthopedic Surgery, Mayo Clinic, Rochester, MN, USA

Scott W. Rogers, MD Department of Orthopaedic Surgery, UPMC Hamot, Erie, PA, USA

Brandon S. Smetana, MD Department of Orthopaedics, University of North Carolina, Chapel Hill, NC, USA

T. Greg Sommerkamp, MD Tri Health- Hand Surgery Specialists, Inc., Crestview Hills, KY, USA

Robert J. Strauch, MD Department of Orthopaedic Surgery, New York-Presbyterian Medical Center, Columbia University, New York, NY, USA

Stephanie Sweet, MD Philadelphia Hand Center, Thomas Jefferson University, King of Prussia, PA, USA

Mark A. Vitale, MD ONS Foundation, Greenwich, CT, USA

Lawrence E. Weiss, MD, Division of Hand Surgery, OAA Hand Center, Lehigh Valley Hospital, Allentown, PA, USA

Terri L. Wolfe, OTR/L, CHT Hand and Upper Body Rehabilitation Center, Erie, PA, USA

Chapter 1
Dorsal Fracture Dislocations: Biomechanics and Management Principles

Brandon S. Smetana and Reid W. Draeger

Abstract Dorsal proximal interphalangeal (PIP) joint fracture dislocations represent difficult injuries to manage and are frequently missed on initial evaluation. During dorsal fracture dislocations of the PIP joint, the volar plate is either disrupted or remains attached to the volar fragments of the middle phalangeal base; thus resistance to dorsal subluxation hinges on the integrity of the bony volar articular buttress of the middle phalanx. Appropriate treatment depends on recognition of dorsal instability, if present, on lateral radiographs and maintenance of reduction throughout the healing process. Anatomic reduction of the articular surface remains less important than maintenance of stability and prevention of dorsal subluxation. As such, the most commonly utilized classification scheme divides these injuries according to the amount of volar middle phalangeal base involved in the fracture dislocation in order to guide treatment. Stable injuries involve less than 30 % of the volar middle phalangeal base and are treated with nonoperative means, typically by buddy taping or with dorsal block splinting. Unstable injuries involve more than 50 % of the volar articular base and necessitate operative intervention

B.S. Smetana, M.D. • R.W. Draeger, M.D. (✉)
Department of Orthopaedics, University of North Carolina,
3102 Bioinformatics Building, CB# 7055, Chapel Hill, NC 27599, USA
e-mail: bsmetana@unch.unc.edu; reid_draeger@med.unc.edu

© Springer International Publishing Switzerland 2016
J.E. Adams (ed.), *PIP Joint Fracture Dislocations*,
DOI 10.1007/978-3-319-28579-5_1

1

to prevent dorsal subluxation. Surgical strategies include open reduction and internal fixation, percutaneous pinning, external fixation, or arthroplasty. Tenuous injuries involve 30–50 % of the volar articular base and appropriate management is less clear.

Keywords Dorsal proximal interphalangeal joint fracture dislocation • Biomechanics • Classification • Treatment • Management principles

Introduction

Finger fractures are common with an annual incidence of 67.9 per 100,000 persons per year with dislocations occurring with an annual incidence of 11.2 per 1000 persons per year [1]. The proximal interphalangeal (PIP) joint sits in an unprotected position and carries a long moment arm, placing it at increased risk of injury compared to surrounding structures [2]. It is additionally susceptible to injury given the high degree of articular congruity between the proximal and middle phalanges [3]. Some injuries to the PIP joint only affect ligamentous structures or are associated with small avulsion fractures of the base of the middle phalanx at the insertion of the palmar plate, while others are associated with larger fractures of the base of the middle phalanx [2]. PIP joint fractures often go unrecognized as "sprains" or "jams" leading to delayed diagnosis. Failure to recognize and treat injuries may result in subsequent stiffness, pain, swelling, angulation, and radiographic changes associated with early arthritis [2]. When dislocations occur in conjunction with fractures, they often are significantly comminuted, can be difficult to treat, and may result in a painful and stiff joint [4]. Although much is written regarding the appropriate management of closed dorsal PIP fracture dislocations, there is wide variation regarding the choice of treatment for these injuries [1, 2, 5]. This chapter reviews the biomechanics of the PIP joint in relation to PIP fracture dislocations and the treatment principles behind the approach to their management.

Biomechanics

Anatomy

The PIP joint is composed of a bicondylar convex proximal phalangeal head with a central groove and a biconcave middle phalangeal articular surface with a central ridge to match the proximal phalanx [6]. The dorsal-volar length of the radial condyles is larger on the index and middle fingers; however the ulnar condyles are larger on the ring and small fingers resulting in the convergence of the fingers toward the volar scaphoid tubercle during flexion [6]. The PIP joint is mostly a simple hinge joint with the majority of motion occurring in the volar/dorsal plane [1, 4], although most refer to it as a "sloppy hinge" due to small amount of rotational and angular motion [1, 7, 8]. The range of motion of the PIP joint averages from 10° of hyperextension to 110° of flexion for a total arc of motion of 100–120° about a static center of rotation [7, 9, 10]. This long arc of motion at the PIP joint contributes to approximately 85 % of finger flexion during grasp [9]. This large range of motion necessitates limited bony constraint with the middle phalangeal articular surface covering approximately 110° of the overall 210° arc of the proximal phalangeal articular surface [10]. The axis of PIP joint rotation is a single static point, which lies on lateral radiographs at an equidistant point from the dorsal, palmar, and distal articular surface of the proximal phalanx [4]. Anatomically, this is found in between the origin of the dorsal and palmar bundles of the proper lateral collateral ligament [4].

Stability of the PIP Joint

Stability of the PIP joint is provided both by the bony architecture of the proximal phalanx head and middle phalangeal base articular surfaces in addition to its soft tissue envelope. Bony constraint is provided by the cup-shaped articular surface of the middle phalangeal base on the cylindrical distal articular surface of the head of

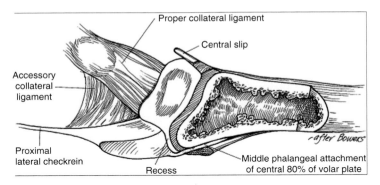

Fig. 1.1 Soft tissue stabilizers of the PIP joint: the "box" configuration. Soft tissue constraint to the PIP joint is afforded by a boxlike configuration composed of four distinct structures surrounding the joint: dorsally the central slip, palmarly the volar plate, and both radially and ulnarly the proper and accessory collateral ligaments (From Williams IV CS. Proximal Interphalangeal Joint Fracture Dislocations: Stable and Unstable. Hand Clinics. 2012; 28:409–416 p.410. Originally published In Bowers WH. The anatomy of the interphalangeal joints. In: Bowers WH, editor. The interphalangeal joints. New York: Churchill Livingstone; 1987. p. 11; with permission)

the proximal phalanx. This bony stability is further enhanced by the central groove separating the radial and ulnar condyles of the proximal phalanx and the corresponding central ridge of the articular surface of the middle phalangeal base.

Soft tissue stability is afforded by a "box" configuration about the hinge joint (Fig. 1.1) [1, 10]. The sides of the box are formed by the radial and ulnar proper and accessory collateral ligaments, the floor by the palmar plate, and the ceiling by the central slip [1]. The palmar plate provides constraint to both hyperextension and dorsal translation of the middle phalanx on the proximal phalanx with intact bony anatomy [10]. It arises from the distal margin of the A2 pulley and inserts at the lateral volar aspect of the middle phalanx [10]. It is composed of thick checkrein portions laterally and a thinner portion centrally [6, 10].

The proper collateral ligaments originate near the center of rotation of the PIP joint at the central aspect of the head of the proximal phalanx and course distally and volarly to insert on the volar proximal aspect of the middle phalangeal base [1, 10]. They act as secondary stabilizers to dorsal translation in addition to providing radial and ulnar stability, especially with the PIP joint in slight flexion [1, 11].

The accessory collateral ligaments are generally less substantial upon anatomical dissection than typically represented on pictorial depictions [1]. They originate from a more distal and volar aspect of the proximal phalanx than the origin of the proper collateral ligaments and course along a more volar trajectory inserting on the volar plate near its insertion [1, 10, 11]. The accessory collateral ligaments help to provide radial and ulnar stability to the PIP joint when in extension.

Injury to the PIP Joint and Instability

Disruption of any one of the soft tissue stabilizers will not typically result in dislocation, as it typically takes injury to at least two of the structures to result in dislocation [1]. With complete disruption of the collateral ligaments and volar plate seen with dislocations, reconstruction is typically not necessary as neocollateral ligaments form and provide adequate stability to the PIP joint [12]. Lutz et al. examined this anatomical ligamentous disruption in a cadaver model during pure dislocation events. In 10° of flexion, reduction of the palmar plate to its insertion occurred, as did reduction of the collateral ligaments to their site of avulsion off of their proximal phalangeal origin [11].

Fractures can commonly occur with dislocation secondary to the transmission of a longitudinally applied force vector and a large angular moment across the joint [2]. Due to variations in force transmission, three different patterns based on the joint position at the time of injury and the injury's force vector are reported (Fig. 1.2): volar lip fractures associated with dorsal fracture dislocations, dorsal lip fractures associated with volar fracture dislocations, and pilon fractures associated with longitudinal load [2]. Hyperextension at the PIP joint leads to either palmar plate disruption near its insertion or volar avulsion injuries of the palmar lip of the middle phalanx, whereas load and shear injuries lead to more profound fractures and comminution [2].

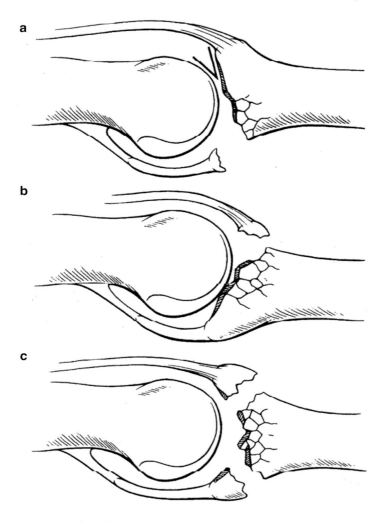

Fig. 1.2 PIP joint fracture dislocation: patterns of injury. (**a**) Palmar lip fracture and dorsal subluxation can arise from either an avulsion (hyperextension)- or an impaction shear (axial load in flexion)-type mechanism. The pattern depicted in this figure represents an impaction shear injury. (**b**) Dorsal lip fracture with palmar subluxation can additionally arise in a similar fashion through avulsion (hyperflexion)- or impaction shear (axial load in relative hyperextension)-type mechanisms. (**c**) Pilon fractures as depicted in this image occur from axial load

When Eaton first classified these injuries, he made reference to a "critical corner" encompassing the palmar plate and lateral collateral ligament attachments to the volar base of the middle phalanx, which, when disrupted, led to instability [2, 13]. He later noted that when greater than 40 % of the palmar articular surface of the middle phalanx was involved that instability resulted secondary to loss of the stabilizing effects of the palmar plate and collateral ligaments [2]. When less is involved, the remaining fibers of the collateral ligament attached to the main middle phalangeal fragment provide adequate palmar stability to prevent dorsal subluxation during extension and subsequent hinging during flexion [2]. Hastings and Carroll further support the biomechanical importance of the volar lip of the middle phalangeal base in preventing dorsal subluxation. They state that when the volar lip fragment becomes of significant size, the normal semicircular shape of the middle phalangeal base is lost leaving behind a small oblique dorsal remnant. This remnant is susceptible to the forces of the central slip in allowing dorsal subluxation about the proximal phalanx [4]. The flexor digitorum superficialis inserting on the middle phalanx additionally creates a rotational moment, exacerbating this apex dorsal deformity, and increases the tendency of the middle phalanx to hinge on the volar articular remnant during flexion [4].

This dorsal subluxation of the middle phalanx necessitates disruption of the continuity of palmar restraints including the volar plate, collateral ligaments, and the palmar bony buttress [14, 15]. The volar plate is invariably disrupted in dorsal dislocations [11], and thus, the primary determinants of stability of PIP joint dorsal fracture dislocations are the degree of volar lip involvement and the subsequent amount of remaining proper collateral ligament fibers attached to the major middle phalangeal fragment [1]. Recent biomechanical evaluation of dorsal fracture dislocations demonstrated uniform stability with involvement of only 20 % of the volar lip and instability with involvement of 60–80 % involvement. 40 % articular

Fig. 1.2 (continued) in extension with disruption of both the dorsal and volar cortical margins (From Kiefhaber TR, Stern PJ. Clinical Perspective: Fracture Dislocations of the Proximal Interphalangeal Joint. Journal of Hand Surgery 1998. 23(A):368–379 p.369. Originally published by Kiefhaber TR. Phalangeal dislocations/periarticular trauma. In: Peimer CA ed. Surgery of the hand and upper extremity. Vol 1. New York: McGraw-Hill, 2996:963; with permission)

involvement had variable amount of instability noted on their evaluation and appeared to be the threshold for stability, although they did not examine 50 % articular involvement [16].

Work by Eaton, Hastings, Carroll, Kiefhaber, and Stern has provided evidence of the importance of the volar lip size in determining stability of the fracture dislocation and provides the basis for PIP joint fracture dislocation management.

Management Principles

Principles of management rest on creating a concentric reduction of the middle and proximal phalanges while avoiding dorsal subluxation of the middle phalanx during terminal extension and subsequent hinging of the middle phalanx during flexion [2, 4]. Poor results have been reported with persistent subluxation [2, 4, 17]. Evidence suggests that the prevention of "hinging" of the PIP articulation is of paramount importance for optimizing PIP fracture dislocation outcomes.

Anatomic reduction of the articular surface is less important for these injuries, as long as concentricity is achieved at the PIP joint. Few investigators and leading clinicians in the field are proponents of joint surface reduction as a main goal of PIP fracture dislocation treatment [2]. There has been increasing evidence that satisfactory outcomes can be obtained without obtaining anatomic articular reduction if joint subluxation is avoided and early motion is instituted [2, 14, 18–20].

Early motion has emerged as a key component of successful management of PIP fracture dislocations and parallels the early work of Salter on the positive impact of continuous passive motion on the cartilage healing process [2, 4, 5, 21]. Although stressed in most reviews, there is a paucity of high-level evidence supporting these claims [1, 2, 4, 5]. A few series claim good outcomes with slightly delayed mobilization (with as much as 3–4 weeks of immobilization) [5], yet some report the contrary with poor outcomes found with a similar period of immobilization [1]. However, with many treatment modalities permitting and demonstrating good results with early active motion, the general consensus rests on instituting motion as early as possible provided that stability is not sacrificed.

Table 1.1 Kiefhaber and Stern's stability-based classification of PIP joint dorsal fracture dislocations

Stable	Tenuous	Unstable
<30 % articular surface involvement	30–50 % articular surface involvement	>50 % articular surface involvement
And	And	Or
Does *not* require >30° of flexion to maintain congruous reduction	Does *not* require >30° of flexion to maintain congruous reduction	Requires >30° of flexion to maintain congruous reduction

Based on the size of the volar lip fragment expressed in percentage of the articular surface and clinical and radiographic stability of the fracture dislocation pattern in terms of amount of flexion required to maintain congruous reduction

Classification

Based on these principles, classifications were developed in hopes of guiding treatment. Eaton first classified PIP fracture dislocations according to degree of injury from a simple hyperextension injury, followed by simple dislocation, to dislocation associated with fracture [13]. He noted the importance of the bony volar aspect of the middle phalanx with instability seen with disruption exceeding 40 % [13]. In a large retrospective series examining injuries to the MCP and PIP joint, Hastings and Carroll additionally stress the importance of the middle phalanx palmar buttress in affording stability to the joint [4]. They found that management of these injuries should center on restoring this buttress and preventing dorsal subluxation [4], which has been confirmed by multiple other investigators [2]. Further investigation has yielded similar findings regarding the importance of the volar lip of the middle phalanx in providing PIP joint stability in the setting of PIP fracture dislocations. It is generally accepted that fractures involving more than 30–40 % of the volar articular base are at risk of dorsal instability [2, 4, 16].

Kiefhaber and Stern noted that not only was the fragment size important in predicting instability, but also examination of dynamic stability was essential in treating these injuries [2]. They proposed a stability-based classification of PIP joint dorsal fracture dislocations based both on fracture size in addition to clinical and radiographic examination of stability. This classification is widely used to guide

Normal

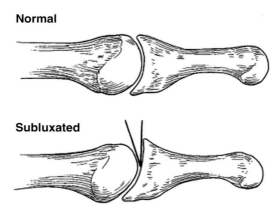

Subluxated

Fig. 1.3 The V-sign: evidence of dorsal subluxation of the middle phalanx. As first described by Light, the V-sign, as seen on a true lateral radiograph of the PIP joint, is an indicator of an otherwise subtle radiographic finding of dorsal subluxation of the middle phalanx on the proximal phalanx after volar injury (From Williams IV CS. Proximal Interphalangeal Joint Fracture Dislocations: Stable and Unstable. Hand Clinics. 2012; 28:409–416 p.410. Originally published by Blazar PE, Steinberg DR. Fractures of the proximal interphalangeal joint. JAAOS. 2000; 8(6): 383–390; with permission)

PIP Fracture Dislocations

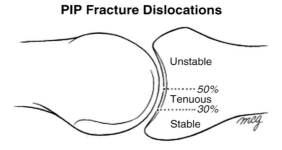

Fig. 1.4 Kiefhaber and Stern's stability-based classification of PIP joint dorsal fracture dislocations: a schematic representation. Within this classification, resultant stability of the PIP joint after dorsal fracture dislocation is classified based on the percentage of joint surface involvement and integrity of the volar articular buttress (From Williams IV CS. Proximal Interphalangeal Joint Fracture Dislocations: Stable and Unstable. Hand Clinics. 2012; 28:409–416 p.410. Originally published by Kiefhaber TR. Phalangeal dislocations/periarticular trauma. In: Peimer CA ed. Surgery of the hand and upper extreity. Vol 1. New York: McGraw-Hill, 2996:963; with permission)

treatment (Table 1.1) [2]. The finger is examined under digital block for clinical signs of subluxation during extension, followed by true lateral radiographic examination in full extension. If subluxation is noted in extension, clinical and radiographic examination with progressive flexion is performed [2]. Many authors additionally stress the importance of recognizing subtle subluxation at the PIP joint on a lateral radiograph by the formation of a "V-sign" first described by Light, between the dorsal distal aspect of the proximal phalanx and the dorsally subluxated articular surface of the middle phalanx (Fig. 1.3) [1, 2, 4, 5, 10]. Based on the clinical and radiographic findings, one may classify PIP fracture dislocations as stable, tenuous, or unstable; a stepwise treatment algorithm is suggested based upon this classification (Fig. 1.4, Table 1.1) [2].

Stable Injuries

Stable injuries about the PIP joint associated with dorsal fracture dislocations represent a range of injuries, from pure hyperextension injuries with small volar avulsion fractures, to fracture dislocations involving less than 30 % of the volar articular base without evidence of joint subluxation at less than 30° of flexion on clinical and true radiographic examination [2]. It is important to examine hyperextension injuries for the presence of persistent hyperextension due to disruption of the palmar plate, as these injuries are prone to developing a swan neck deformity. Additionally, when stable volar fractures are present, the degree of flexion necessary to obtain concentric reduction is important, as this will guide initial degree of permitted extension during early motion rehabilitation protocol. In the setting of hyperextensibility or with subluxation seen near terminal extension, treatment with extension block splinting [22], figure-of-eight bracing, short-arm casting with dorsal extension block, or a double AlumaFoam splint according to Strong's method [23] can be utilized to allow for full flexion but prevent hyperextension, while the palmar stabilizing structures heal [2]. Similarly, a transarticular K-wire extending from the distal aspect of the proximal phalangeal articular surface, serving as a PIP extension block, may be utilized while allowing early motion and avoiding problems with noncompliance with splint wear [1, 2, 4].

If the injury does not result in any clinical hyperextension or sub-luxation with terminal extension, then simple buddy taping is usually sufficient to allow institution of early, unrestricted motion [2]. Early motion is critical in the management of these injuries, and prolonged immobilization in lieu of dorsal block splinting or buddy taping is not advised due to problems with stiffness and development of flexion contractures [2].

Tenuous Injuries

Tenuous injuries consist of those involving 30–50 % of the volar articular surface of the PIP joint, which also demonstrate concentric reduction with less than 30° of flexion [2]. In this scenario, close observation is critical, as joint reduction and stability must be maintained until fracture union and soft tissue stability are achieved. Typically, dorsal block splinting as described above is performed for fractures fitting this description with gradual increase in extension over a course of 6–8 weeks with close clinical and radiographic examination for evidence of subluxation with a low threshold to transition to operative intervention [2]. However, limited data exists promoting either nonoperative or operative intervention of these injuries falling into this category. If at any point greater than 30° of flexion is necessary to provide stable reduction, the injury should be reclassifed as "unstable" and surgical intervention should be entertained [2]. Tenuous injuries requiring >30° of flexion to maintain concentric reduction are thought to be associated with a greater tendency to subluxate with nonoperative treatment protocols. Additionally, greater stiffness, pain, and flex-ion contracture development may be associated with prolonged immobilization at >30° of flexion.

Unstable Injuries

Unstable injuries are those with fractures involving greater than 50 % of the articular surface or those in which greater than 30° of PIP flexion is required to maintain joint congruity. In these scenarios, operative intervention is indicated to restore the volar buttress and permit early motion without hinging, in order to avoid stiffness, degenerative changes, and flexion contracture associated with nonoperative management and persistent subluxation [2]. Many various operative techniques and interventions are described, and evidence is lacking to demonstrate superiority of one intervention over the others. Review of case series reports on various treatment techniques yields no consistent difference in outcome measures between the performed procedures including joint range of motion, flexion contracture, radiographic changes at final follow-up, or pain [5]. Commonly performed and utilized treatments include longitudinal traction devices (Schenck) [24], closed reduction and K-wire fixation, closed reduction and external fixation, ORIF using small screws or K-wire fixation, tension banding, palmar plate arthroplasty as pioneered by Malerich and Eaton [25], and hemi-hamate arthroplasty [2, 4, 26]. Numerous external fixator designs, such as Agee's force couple [18] utilizing a palmarly directed force to ensure maintenance of joint reduction, custom external fixator about the center of rotation of the PIP joint [4], dynamic external fixators [20, 27], and the Suzuki design [28], have all been developed and promoted with similar results. Successful surgical intervention typically results in an arc of motion between 65 and 90°, with flexion contractures of up to 25°. Reports have shown that patients tolerate 15–20° flexion contractures without functional deficit and their incidence does not significantly differ across techniques [3].

Chronic dorsal fracture dislocations should be considered a distinct entity from acute injuries, as approach and treatment differ substantially. Hinging of the volar remnant articular middle phalangeal base limits flexion arc, and, if left untreated, erosion at this location ensues due to focal increased contact pressure. Determining the amount of joint erosion and degenerative changes about the nonreduced fragments is essential to determining the potential success or failure of an attempted reduction and stabilization procedure. If significant erosion or degenerative changes exist, reduction should be avoided as this will likely result in residual pain, and arthrodesis or arthroplasty should instead be entertained [2]. If reduction of a chronic dislocation is performed, release of the dorsal soft tissue adhesions and augmentation of the

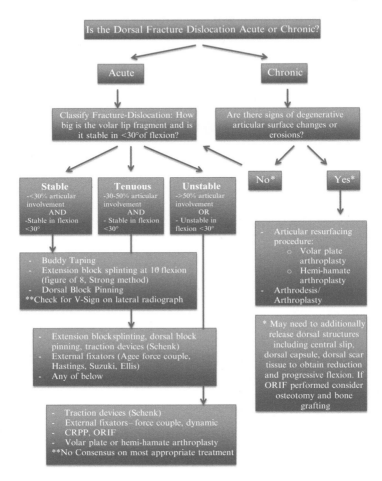

Fig. 1.5 Treatment algorithm for managing dorsal fracture dislocations of the PIP joint

volar restrains with flexor digitorum superficialis tendon slips and/or osteotomy with bone grafting are often necessary [2]. Alternatively, performing palmar plate arthroplasty [2] or hemi-hamate arthroplasty [26] have emerged as successful alternatives to more traditional approaches. Advantages of performing palmar plate or hemi-hamate arthroplasty involve restoring the palmar buttress and tightening volar structures while providing smooth gliding surface.

A treatment algorithm based on Kiefhaber and Stern's stability-based classification and the abovementioned treatment options can be seen in Fig. 1.5.

Conclusions

The volar articular surface of the middle phalangeal base represents the main stabilizing structure after a dorsal PIP joint dislocation. Appropriate initial evaluation of dorsal PIP fracture dislocations rests on determining the degree of involvement of the volar middle phalangeal base and identifying the subsequent presence or absence of dorsal subluxation on a true lateral radiograph. Treatment is instituted to maintain concentric reduction via nonoperative or operative means based on stability of the injury pattern, and many modalities exist to accomplish this goal. Further investigation would be valuable to compare outcomes between analogous treatment options in order to determine optimal treatment algorithms.

References

1. Haase SC, Chung KC. Current concepts in treatment of fracture-dislocations of the proximal interphalangeal joint. J Plast Reconstr Surg. 2014;134:1246–57.
2. Kiefhaber TR, Stern PJ. Fracture dislocations of the proximal interphalangeal joint. J Hand Surg. 1998;23A(3):368–79.
3. Mangelson JJ, Stern PJ, Abzug JM, Chang J, Osterman AL. Complications following dislocations of the proximal interphalangeal joint. Instr Course Lect. 2014;63:123–30.
4. Hastings II H, Carroll IV C. Treatment of closed articular fractures of the metacarpophalangeal and proximal interphalangeal joints. Hand Clin. 1988;4(3):503–27.
5. McAuliffe JA. Dorsal fracture dislocation of the proximal interphalangeal joint. J Hand Surg. 2008;33(10):1885–8.

6. Khouri JS, Bloom JMP, Hammert WC. Current trends in the management of proximal interphalangeal joint injuries of the hand. J Plast Reconstr Surg. 2013;132:1192–204.

7. Leijnse JNAL, Quesada PM, Spoor CW. Kinematic evaluation of the finger's interphalangeal joints coupling mechanism – variability, flexion-extension differences, triggers, locking, swanneck deformities, anthropometric correlations. J Biomech. 2010;43:2381–93.

8. Uchiyama S, Cooney III P, Linscheid RL, Niebur G, An KN. Kinematics of the proximal interphalangeal joint of the finger after surface replacement. J Hand Surg. 2000;25(A):305–12.

9. Liebovic SJ. Anatomy of the proximal interphalangeal joint. Hand Clin. 1994;10:169–78.

10. Williams IV CS. Proximal interphalangeal joint fracture dislocations stable and unstable. Hand Clin. 2012;28:409–16.

11. Lutz M, Fritz D, Arora R, Kathrein A, Gabl M, Pechlaner S, Del Frari B, Poisel S. Anatomical basis for functional treatment of dorsolateral dislocation of the proximal interphalangeal joint. Clin Anat. 2004;17:303–7.

12. Eaton RF, Sunde D, Pang D, Singson R. Evaluation of "neocollateral" ligament formation by magnetic resonance imaging after total excision of the proximal interphalangeal collateral ligaments. J Hand Surg. 1998;23: 322–7.

13. Eaton RG. Joint injuries of the hand. Springfield, IL: Charles C. Thomas; 1971. p. 9–34.

14. Deitch MA, Kiefhaber TR, Comisar BR, Stern PJ. Dorsal fracture dislocations of the proximal interphalangeal joint: surgical complications and long-term results. J Hand Surg. 1999;24(A):914–23.

15. Lee JYL, Teoh LC. Dorsal fracture dislocations of the proximal interphalangeal joint treated by open reduction and interfragmentary screw fixation: indications, approaches, and results. J Hand Surg Br. 2006;31(B):138–46.

16. Tyser AR, Tsai MA, Parks BG, Means Jr KR. Stability of acute dorsal fracture dislocations of the proximal interphalangeal joint: a biomechanical study. J Hand Surg. 2014;39:13–8.

17. Hamer DW, Quinton DN. Dorsal fracture subluxation of the proximal interphalangeal joints treated by extension block splintage. J Hand Surg. 1992;17(B):586–90.

18. Agee JM. Unstable fracture dislocations of the proximal interphalangeal joint. Treatment with the force couple splint. Clin Orthop. 1987;214: 101–12.

19. Morgan JP, Gordon DA, Klug MS, Perry PE, Barre PS. Dynamic digital traction for unstable comminuted intraarticular fracture-dislocations of the proximal interphalangeal joint. J Hand Surg. 1995;20(A):565–73.

20. Ellis SJ, Chen R, Prokopis P, Chetboun A, Wolfe SW, Athanasian EA, Weiland AJ. Treatment of proximal interphalangeal dorsal fracture-dislocation injuries with dynamic external fixation: a pins and rubber band system. J Hand Surg. 2007;32A(8):1242–50.

21. Salter RB. The physiologic basis of continuous passive motion for articular cartilage healing and regeneration. Hand Clin. 1994;10:211–20.
22. McElFresh EC, Dobyns JH, O'Brien ET. Management of fracture-dislocation of the proximal interphalangeal joints by extension-block splinting. J Bone Joint Surg Am. 1972;54(A):1705–11.
23. Strong ML. A new method of extension block splinting for the proximal interphalangeal joint – preliminary report. J Hand Surg. 1980;7(A):77–8.
24. Schenck RR. Dynamic traction and early passive movement for fractures for the proximal interphalangeal joint. J Hand Surg. 1986;11(A):850–8.
25. Malerich MM, Eaton RG. The volar plate reconstruction for fracture-dislocation of the proximal interphalangeal joint. Hand Clin. 1994;10:251–60.
26. Williams RM, Hastings II H, Kiefhaber TR. PIP fracture/dislocation treatment technique: use of a hemi-hamate resurfacing arthroplasty. Tech Hand Up Extrem Surg. 2002;6(4):185–92.
27. Ruland RT, Hogan CJ, Cannon DL, Slade JF. Use of dynamic distraction external fixation for unstable fracture-dislocations of the proximal interphalangeal joint. J Hand Surg. 2008;33(1):19–25.
28. Suzuki Y, Matsunaga T, Sato S, Yoki Y. The pins and rubber traction system for treatment of comminuted intraarticular fractures and fracture-dislocations in the hand. J Hand Surg. 1994;19(B):98–107.

Chapter 2
Dorsal Block Splinting for Dorsal Fracture-Dislocations

C. Liam Dwyer, Scott W. Rogers, Alex J. Ferikes,
John D. Lubahn, Terri L. Wolfe, and Katie Froehlich

Abstract There are a variety of treatment options for dorsal fracture-dislocations of the proximal interphalangeal (PIP) joint. Extension block splinting is a form of nonoperative management that focuses on maintaining an acceptable reduction of the PIP joint while allowing for adequate, safe motion. By maintaining a reduced joint, the extension block orthosis allows the ligamentous structures surrounding the PIP joint to heal in their anatomic locations. The risk of developing a flexion contracture, which is high with any PIP joint injury, is minimized with the use of an extension block orthosis because of its ability to allow early active motion of the PIP joint while controlling PIPJ flexion. This chapter describes a clinical case utilizing extension block splinting for a dorsal fracture-dislocation of the PIP joint.

C.L. Dwyer, M.D. • S.W. Rogers, M.D. • A.J. Ferikes, M.D.
J.D. Lubahn, M.D.
Department of Orthopaedic Surgery, UPMC Hamot,
201 State Street, Erie, PA 16550, USA
e-mail: c.liam.dwyer@gmail.com; scottie_rog@hotmail.com;
ferikes@gmail.com; jdlubahn@jdlubahn.com

T.L. Wolfe, O.T.R./L., C.H.T. (✉) • K. Froehlich, O.T.R./L., C.H.T.
Hand and Upper Body Rehabilitation Center, 300 State Street,
Erie, PA 16507, USA
e-mail: TerriWolfe@eriehandcenter.com; Froehlichk8@gmail.com

© Springer International Publishing Switzerland 2016
J.E. Adams (ed.), *PIP Joint Fracture Dislocations*,
DOI 10.1007/978-3-319-28579-5_2

Keywords Dorsal block orthosis • Dorsal • Proximal interphalangeal joint • Fracture-dislocation

Introduction

Although there are general guidelines regarding the treatment options for dorsal PIP joint dislocations, the decision-making algorithm greatly depends on surgeon preference, experience, and clinical judgment. The risk of stiffness with PIP joint injuries is high; therefore early diagnosis and management with active range of motion while maintaining joint stability is critical to obtaining quality results [3]. The key benefit of *extension block splinting* as a treatment option is that it is a nonoperative treatment option that allows for early motion thereby minimizing the risk of a contracture.

Case History

A 33-year-old woman fell as she was entering the shower and noted immediate pain and deformity in both the long and ring fingers of her left hand. She presented later that day to a local emergency room where an exam was suspicious for dorsal dislocations of the PIPJs of the long and ring fingers. Radiographs confirmed the fracture-dislocations. A closed reduction of both digits was performed under digital block anesthesia, and post-reduction X-rays were satisfactory with small avulsion fractures of the palmar plate insertion in the base of the middle phalanx of both fingers. Her collateral ligaments were felt to be stable, and after a discussion with the hand surgeon on call, she was placed in a static dorsal AlumaFoam® orthosis for each finger with the PIPJs held in 30° of flexion and asked to see a hand surgeon a few days later.

Physical Exam Findings

When evaluated in the clinic 3 days later, moderate swelling and ecchymosis was noted in each of the fingers.

Tenderness was noted upon palpation of the collateral ligaments of both the long and ring fingers and active flexion in the PIPJ of both fingers was from 30 to 60°. No instability could be demonstrated in the PIPJ of either injured finger. Radiographs confirmed a stable, congruent reduction of both fingers with a small avulsion fragment at the palmar plate insertion in the base of the middle phalanx of the long finger.

Because the patient had a stable (<30 % of joint surface fracture) and concentric reduction with flexion of the digit to 30°, she was felt to be a good candidate for extension block splinting as a treatment option. The patient was then referred to a certified hand therapist (CHT) with a prescription for an extension block orthosis in 30° of flexion for the long and ring fingers.

Treatment Options

The stability of dorsal fracture-dislocations of the PIP joint is a key in determining the required treatment. Stability can be predicted based on the amount or percentage of middle phalanx articular surface involved [5]. While the ranges of involvement, <30 % considered stable, 30–50 % considered tenuous, and >50 % considered unstable [6], are useful reference points, joint stability must be determined clinically by physical exam during treatment [7]. During physical examination, the amount of extension allowable while maintaining stability may be ascertained. Typically, there is increased stability with greater amounts of flexion, and if a patient requires more than 30° of flexion to remain reduced, the injury is determined to be unstable [4]. The best time to determine stability is immediately following PIPJ reduction. With the digital block still functioning, radial and ulnar collateral ligament stability is checked in varying degrees of PIPJ flexion. The finger is also passively extended until instability is demonstrated and the amount of extension to create instability is noted.

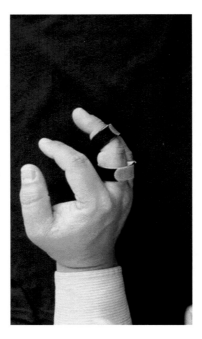

Fig. 2.1 Buddy taping to noninvolved digit

Stable injuries and tenuous injuries without hinging may be treated closed with buddy taping (Fig. 2.1) or extension block splinting (Fig. 2.2) while allowing for motion and function to be restored [7–9]. Allowing for active mobilization of the joint has shown to provide superior results to static immobilization [8, 10]. Unstable injuries, on the other hand, require surgical management and represent a contraindication to the use of extension block splinting [9].

Treatment Chosen

Initially described by McElfresh et al. [7], a dorsal orthosis to block proximal interphalangeal joint extension was selected for this patient (Fig. 2.2). This method remained a viable option as the PIP

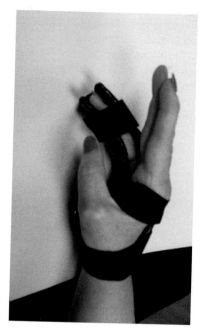

Fig. 2.2   Extension block orthosis with flexion at PIP joint to protect against re-dislocation

joint was able to be maintained in a reduced position in the orthosis [9]. The benefit of the extension block orthosis is that it permits motion in the stable range in efforts to prevent flexion contracture unlike static immobilization in a flexed position [15, 16].

Although acceptable outcomes have been described with treatment of immobilization in 50–60° flexion [7], surgical management is generally advocated if greater than 30° flexion is required to maintain reduction in order to optimize results [1, 4]. These general recommendations are made without high level of evidence studies reporting defined guidelines for unstable PIP joint fracture-dislocations to be treated nonoperatively, specifically in regard to the flexion required for stability. Given that Lutz et al. [16] demonstrated appropriate anatomic realignment of the palmar plate and collateral ligaments about the PIP joint after reduction of dorsolateral dislocations in a cadaveric study, it appears that, as long as the PIP joint is held in a reduced position while allowing enough motion to limit flexion contracture, nonoperative treatment will have satisfactory results. This is supported in that the restoration of the joint surface may not hold clinical significance as articular step-off, gap, or depression does not have a negative impact on range of motion, pain, or patient satisfaction [11–15].

If joint stability and concentric PIP joint reduction are maintained and the patient can understand and is cooperative, then an extension block nonoperative program can be advised.

Hand Therapy/Post Injury/Postoperatively

Patient outcomes are improved when the patient is referred to a certified hand therapist with a prescription clearly stating the diagnosis and recommended therapy. For example, the diagnosis should read: "dorsal PIPJ dislocation orthosis in 30° of flexion at the PIPJ with gradual extension over 3 weeks to neutral or 0°."

A team approach to hand injuries includes having the patient become a member of the team in order to better understand treatment and recovery time and a patient's personal commitment to exercise and use his/her orthosis. Having the therapist and the surgeon meet however briefly with the patient helps convey the importance of a team approach and the importance of having the patient on the same team is critical. Furthermore, the patient is made to feel that he or she is responsible for the final outcome and that adherence to the postoperative protocol or post-injury protocol is critical to obtaining a successful outcome. The therapist and patient can then develop a plan of care, which allows for active and passive range of motion which is appropriate for the extent of the injury sustained. A certified hand therapist understands the pathophysiology and biomechanics of the injury as well as time to healing and knows to consult the surgeon if increased swelling or loss of motion occurs.

The first stage of treatment should be to protect the injured joint. The therapist should know whether or not there is a fracture fragment from the middle phalanx attached to the palmar plate. After 1 or 2 days of static splinting, motion can be started in an extension block orthosis with the PIPJ held in 25–30° of flexion. The physician deter-

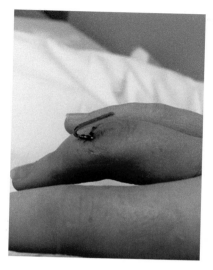

Fig. 2.3   Pinning of dorsal dislocation

mines the amount of flexion based on stability of the PIPJ post reduction. In patients that are treated with an extension block pin or K-wire, the orthosis is used to cover the pin for protection and may be removed to allow active PIPJ extension against the K-wire (Fig. 2.3). In patients with other associated injuries, or more severe injuries, a forearm-based orthosis (Fig. 2.4) extending on to the finger as an extension block may be considered. In the static orthosis, the middle phalanx is held to the orthosis with tape or a Velcro strap. This strap is removed to allow active flexion of the PIPJ.

   Current practice supports early motion even with mildly unstable injuries. The benefits of early motion outweigh the risks, and the results of early protected motion are improved soft tissue healing, better tendon excursion, and improved joint mobility. It is important to avoid prolonged immobilization which leads to joint stiffness, pain, and degenerative changes with poor long-term results. Ideally, all treatment is based on evidence-based research; however, little exists on the benefits of early motion in fracture-dislocations of the PIPJ. There is evidence, however, to support early active and/or passive motion in any fracture or ligamentous injury to improve nutrition

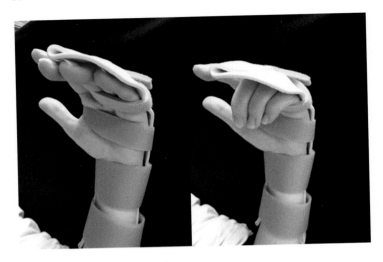

Fig. 2.4 Forearm-based orthosis

of the articular cartilage and ultimately to achieve better motion and overall function [18]. Typically, dorsal fracture-dislocation of the PIPJ can begin motion immediately as long as they are maintained in an extension block orthosis to prevent hyperextension and re-dislocation. Once the volar plate has healed, usually between 3 and 4 weeks, transition to buddy taping the injured finger to the adjacent, non-injured finger may begin. Care should be taken to protect any collateral ligament injury, for example, if the radial collateral ligament of the middle finger is torn, buddy tape should be with the index finger. If the ulnar collateral ligament of the middle finger is involved, buddy tape should be to the ring finger.

Clinical Problems and Solutions

More attention by a therapist may be required if the patient begins to lose PIPJ motion, develops a PIPJ hyperextension (swan neck deformity), or the oblique retinacular ligament tightness.

The surgeon and therapist should be aware of the potential to develop a pseudo-boutonniere deformity. This is basically a flexion contracture of the PIPJ with what appears to be hyperextension of the

DIPJ. When the PIPJ is flexed, however, there is no evidence of tightness of the ORL and the DIPJ can be flexed without difficulty.

Reverse blocking exercises are the most effective method to gain active extension at the PIPJ, especially when full passive PIPJ extension can be achieved. The MPJ is held in flexion to direct the pull of the EDC more distal. This can be done manually, with an item such as a pen (Fig. 2.5), or with the aid of a reverse blocking orthosis.

Relative motion (RM) orthosis (Fig. 2.6) has been described by Howell [19]. The orthotic holds the adjacent joints to be more extended at the MCPJ than the finger with limited motion (the dislocated PIPJ). MCPJ flexion and AROM at the PIPJ are allowed. The PIPJ is cradled in passive extension while avoiding hyperextension.

Hyperextension at the PIPJ (swan neck deformity) may be treated with a static orthosis with slight (30°) flexion. This can be functional during the day to allow motion or remain static at night to keep the PIPJ

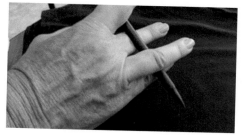

Fig. 2.5   Use of a pen to perform reverse blocking exercise for maximal active PIP extension

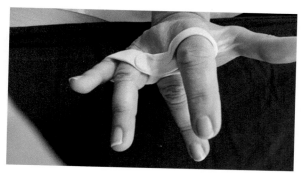

Fig. 2.6   Relative motion (RM) orthosis

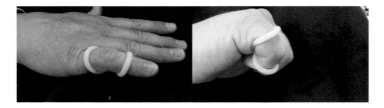

Fig. 2.7 Prefabricated figure of 8 orthosis

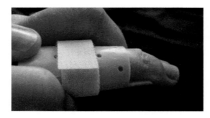

Fig. 2.8 Orthosis to stabilize PIP in extension to achieve DIP active motion

in flexion. A blocking orthosis that holds the MPJ and DIPJ in static position allows focus of motion at the PIPJ. A custom or prefabricated figure of 8 orthosis (Fig. 2.7) can be very effective by providing 3-point fixation and limiting PIPJ hyperextension during daily activities.

Oblique retinacular ligament tightness can be addressed by holding the PIPJ in extension, once stability allows, and passively flexing the DIPJ. Early DIP blocking exercises may prevent ORL tightness, pending fracture stability, and integrity of the lateral bands. This can be effectively treated with a static orthosis (Fig. 2.8) or cylinder cast to allow DIPJ flexion while holding the PIPJ extended.

Several variations of the abovementioned orthoses can be fabricated according to the individual need of the patient (Fig. 2.9).

Summary

Early diagnosis and timely management are critical in the treatment of dorsal fracture-dislocations of the PIP joint. There are a variety of nonsurgical and operative techniques to select from depending on the injury characteristics, patient factors, and surgeon preference.

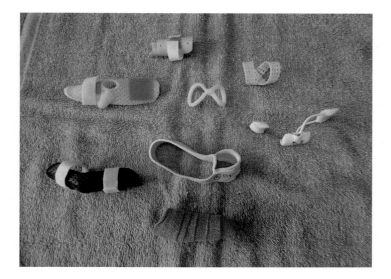

Fig. 2.9 Splinting options for PIP joint

The goals of establishing a well-aligned, reduced joint with satis-factory motion and pain-free function remain the same across all treatment options. While PIP joint fracture-dislocations inherently lead to some acceptable loss of motion [2], nonoperative treatment using an extension block splinting protocol for select injuries results in satisfactory outcomes.

References

1. Green DP. Green's operative hand surgery. 6th ed. Philadelphia, PA: Churchill Livingstone; 2005.
2. Elfar J, Mann T. Fracture-dislocations of the proximal interphalangeal joint. J Am Acad Orthop Surg. 2013;21:88–98. doi:10.5435/JAAOS-21-02-88.
3. Strickland JW, Steichen JB, American Society for Surgery of the Hand. Difficult problems in hand surgery. St. Louis, MO: Mosby; 1982. xiii, 434.
4. Kiefhaber TR. Phalangeal dislocations/periarticular trauma. New York, NY: McGraw-Hill Professional Publishing; 1996.
5. Hastings 2nd H, Carroll 4th C. Treatment of closed articular fractures of the metacarpophalangeal and proximal interphalangeal joints. Hand Clin. 1988;4:503–27.

6. McAuliffe JA. Dorsal fracture dislocation of the proximal interphalangeal joint. J Hand Surg [Am]. 2008;33:1885–8. doi:10.1016/j.jhsa.2008.08.017.

7. McElfresh EC, Dobyns JH, O'Brien ET. Management of fracture-dislocation of the proximal interphalangeal joints by extension-block splinting. J Bone Joint Surg Am. 1972;54:1705–11.

8. Phair IC, Quinton DN, Allen MJ. The conservative management of volar avulsion fractures of the P.I.P. joint. J Hand Surg (Br). 1989;14:168–70. doi:10.1016/0266-7681(89)90120-4.

9. Hamer DW, Quinton DN. Dorsal fracture subluxation of the proximal interphalangeal joints treated by extension block splintage. J Hand Surg (Br). 1992;17:586–90. doi:10.1016/S0266-7681(05)80249-9.

10. Arora R, Lutz M, Fritz D, Zimmermann R, Gabl M, Pechlaner S. Dorsolateral dislocation of the proximal interphalangeal joint: closed reduction and early active motion or static splinting; a retrospective study. Arch Orthop Trauma Surg. 2004;124:486–8. doi:10.1007/s00402-004-0707-0.

11. Newington DP, Davis TR, Barton NJ. The treatment of dorsal fracture-dislocation of the proximal interphalangeal joint by closed reduction and Kirschner wire fixation: a 16-year follow up. J Hand Surg (Br). 2001;26:537–40. doi:10.1054/jhsb.2001.0698.

12. Duteille F, Pasquier P, Lim A, Dautel G. Treatment of complex interphalangeal joint fractures with dynamic external traction: a series of 20 cases. Plast Reconstr Surg. 2003;111:1623–9. doi:10.1097/01.PRS.0000054160.46502.D0.

13. Majumder S, Peck F, Watson JS, Lees VC. Lessons learned from the management of complex intra-articular fractures at the base of the middle phalanges of fingers. J Hand Surg (Br). 2003;28:559–65. doi:10.1016/S0266-7681(03)00139-6.

14. Dionysian E, Eaton RG. The long-term outcome of volar plate arthroplasty of the proximal interphalangeal joint. J Hand Surg [Am]. 2000;25:429–37. doi:10.1016/S0363-5023(00)70026-8.

15. Kuczynski K. The proximal interphalangeal joint. Anatomy and causes of stiffness in the fingers. J Bone Joint Surg (Br). 1968;50:656–63.

16. Lutz M, Fritz D, Arora R, Kathrein A, Gabl M, Pechlaner S, Del Frari B, Poisel S. Anatomical basis for functional treatment of dorsolateral dislocation of the proximal interphalangeal joint. Clin Anat. 2004;17:303–7. doi:10.1002/ca.10216.

17. Deitch MA, Kiefhaber TR, Comisar BR, Stern PJ. Dorsal fracture dislocations of the proximal interphalangeal joint: surgical complications and long-term results. J Hand Surg [Am]. 1999;24:914–23. doi:10.1053/jhsu.1999.0914.

18. Salter RB, Simmonds DF, Malcolm BW, Rumble EJ, MacMichael D, Clements ND. The biological effect of continuous passive motion on the healing of full-thickness defects in articular cartilage. An experimental investigation in the rabbit. J Bone Joint Surg Am. 1980;62:1232–51.

19. Howell JW, Merritt WH, Robinson SJ. Immediate controlled active motion following zone 4-7 extensor tendon repair. J Hand Ther. 2005;18:182–90. doi:10.1197/j.jht.2005.02.011.

Chapter 3
Dorsal Block Pinning

Erica J. Gauger and Julie E. Adams

Abstract   Proximal interphalangeal joint fracture-dislocations are common injuries usually resulting from a direct axial force applied to the tip of the finger. This chapter will focus on describing the indications and the technique for dorsal extension block pinning. This technique is simple, inexpensive, and straightforward. It allows the soft tissue structures to heal, while the joint reduction is maintained in a congruent fashion and motion is permitted in the stable arc. This technique is ideal for the PIP joint injury in which a closed reduction can be obtained, but is unstable. It allows for the advantages of dorsal block splinting without the technical and compliance challenges of fitting a splint and maintaining it in place.

Keywords   Proximal interphalangeal joint • Fracture • Dislocation • Extension block pinning

E.J. Gauger, M.D.
University of Minnesota Medical Center,
2450 Riverside Ave R 200, Minneapolis, MN 55454, USA

J.E. Adams, M.D. (✉)
Mayo Clinic, 1000 1st Ave NW, Austin, MN 55912, USA
e-mail: adams.julie.e@gmail.com

© Springer International Publishing Switzerland 2016   31
J.E. Adams (ed.), *PIP Joint Fracture Dislocations*,
DOI 10.1007/978-3-319-28579-5_3

Introduction

Injuries to the proximal interphalangeal joint (PIPJ) are common-place and most often the result of a direct force applied to the fingertip with axial loading and/or hyperextension across the joint [1, 2]. The severity of these injuries is often underestimated initially and can lead to misdiagnosis or delay in treatment, ultimately leading to poorer outcomes [3]. Potential complications associated with PIPJ fracture-dislocations include stiffness, persistent pain, recurrent instability, and degenerative arthritis [4]. The main goals of treatment are to achieve a stable proximal interphalangeal joint with a functional range of motion and minimal pain and dysfunction.

Treatment of PIPJ fracture-dislocations can be challenging. This chapter will focus specifically on the technique of dorsal, or extension, block pinning.

Pathoanatomy

The most common pattern of fracture-dislocation of the PIPJ includes a fracture through the volar base of the middle phalanx that allows the remainder of the middle phalanx to subluxate or dislocate dorsally with respect to the proximal phalanx. The PIPJ has a degree of inherent bony stability due to the shape of the proximal and middle phalanges. Soft tissue structures which also contribute to stability include the radial and ulnar collateral ligaments, volar plate, dorsal capsule, lateral bands, central tendon of the dorsal apparatus, and flexor tendon sheath [2]. Following an injury, the stability of the joint after reduction is largely dependent on the size of the fractured fragment.

Generally, as described in previous chapters, if the volar fracture fragment is less than 30 % of the articular surface, a concentric reduction can be obtained and maintained via closed nonoperative methods. When the volar fragment is greater than 30–40 % of the articular surface, there is a strong likelihood of persistent instability after reduction [5]. This is due to the attachment site of the true collateral ligaments such that when the fracture is <30 % of the articular surface, some of the attachment remains on the intact middle phalanx. When the fracture is >40 %, it is more likely that the entire collateral ligament is attached to the fractured piece, leading to greater instability of the remaining middle phalanx. When this is the case, surgical intervention is often needed in order to restore a stable joint. Extension block pinning is suited for the patient in whom a closed reduction of the PIPJ can be obtained but is unstable. The ideal patient is one in whom the joint remains congruently reduced in less than 30 or 40° of flexion.

Treatment

Ed McElfresh originally described the technique of extension block splinting in 1972. This technique involves a reduction of the fracture-dislocation and then assessment under fluoroscopy to determine the stable arc of motion. The PIPJ is then held in 10–20° additional flexion from the point where it started to subluxate. Patients are allowed active range of motion within the confines of the splint. The degree of extension allowed is slowly increased over time until splinting is discontinued [6]. This technique is effective; however the splinting can be cumbersome and requires a compliant patient. Additionally, McElfresh and Dobyns recommended this treatment for patients with fractures of 30 % or less of the articular surface and some patients with fractures 30–50 %, although they stated that surgical intervention needed to be considered in those patients.

In order to avoid the cumbersome splint and to remove the concerns of compliance with splint usage, the technique of dorsal block pinning was introduced. Sugawa originally described the technique in 1979 under the principle that the extension block provided by the K-wire prevented compressive loads across the volar base of the middle phalanx. This not only prevented repeat dorsal subluxation or dislocation, but also eliminated the need for permanent fracture fixation or bone graft to support the reduction [7].

Surgical Technique

This technique involves placing a 0.045–0.054 in. smooth K-wire dorsally through the head of the proximal phalanx, preventing terminal extension (Fig. 3.1). This is placed with a minidriver under power and is ideally placed adjacent to the extensor apparatus to avoid piercing the extensor tendon and creating adhesions. Position of the pin is checked with intraoperative fluoroscopy. This wire allows the finger to move through a full arc of flexion but prevents terminal extension of approximately 30–40° short of full extension, therefore preventing it from extending into a position of risk for repeat subluxation or dislocation [8, 9]. The joint should then be brought through a range of motion under fluoroscopy to verify that the joint remains congruently reduced throughout a full arc of motion (as permitted by the dorsal K-wire). If satisfactory reduction is maintained, the K-wire can be trimmed to length and left outside the skin.

Supervised hand therapy is initiated immediately to allow full active flexion and extension as limited by the wire. The wire is left protruding and usually removed 3–4 weeks postoperatively if radiographs confirm maintenance of reduction. Active flexion of the joint is allowed and is encouraged while the wire is in place. The patient works closely with the therapist in order to ensure range of motion is returning. After pin removal the patient continues work with the therapist, to focus on regaining terminal extension.

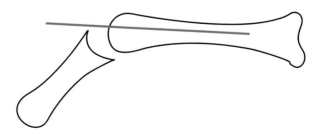

Fig. 3.1 Drawing schematic demonstrating conceptually dorsal block pinning. The pin is placed through the head of the proximal phalanx (eccentrically to avoid piercing the extensor apparatus) in a fashion to prevent terminal extension

Results

Several authors have written about this technique with satisfactory results and minimal complications [7–11]. Viegas in 1992 described using dorsal block pinning in three cases of PIPJ fracture-dislocation with the fracture fragment involving 35–75 % of the articular surface. A single smooth K-wire was placed into the dorsal distal aspect of the proximal phalanx allowing full flexion of the PIPJ but blocking the last 30° of extension. The wires were removed at 4 weeks, and generally by 8 weeks postoperatively, the patients had regained full or near full extension and an average of 110° of flexion. The third patient in the series did not return for follow-up after his wire was removed. There were no major complication and no infections. One patient required reduction of an impacted fracture fragment with an intramedullary K-wire in the middle phalanx that was used for reduction and then removed prior to the end of the operation [9].

Inoue and Tamura in 1991 reported on the use of an extension block K-wire in a series of 14 patients with PIPJ fracture-dislocations. In three patients, the fracture involved less than 30 % of the articular surface and in 11 patients it involved more than 30 %. Four patients had fractures greater than 50 % of the articular surface. All were treated with either closed or open reduction, fracture fixation as needed as well as the placement of an extension block K-wire. The extension block wire was placed with the PIPJ in 30–40° of flexion and was placed on either side of the extensor apparatus. Active flexion was allowed immediately following surgery. The K-wire was removed at 3 weeks and progressive mobilization was permitted. At an average follow-up of 14 months, the average PIPJ range of motion was 94°. In general, the authors report that full flexion is gained by 6 weeks postoperatively, but full extension is not regained until 8–16 weeks postoperatively [11].

Waris and Alanen described a method of percutaneous reduction in addition to dorsal block pinning for these injuries, with the rationale that dorsal block pinning alone does not restore the congruency of the articular surface [10]. Dorsal block pinning was performed as previously described [9]. If an articular step off remained, they then performed percutaneous intramedullary reduction of the fracture fragment to help restore the congruency of the articular surface. This was done with a pre-bent K-wire inserted through a 2 mm percutaneous hole in the lateral distal middle phalanx, volar to the extensor tendon, which was then used to disimpact the fracture fragment. The wire was removed prior to the end of the surgical procedure. The fractures in this series averaged 53 % of the articular surface.

The authors reported on 13 patients, 15 fingers, with an average follow-up time of 5 years. At final follow-up, the average PIPJ motion was 83° with a 3° flexion contracture. Six of 15 fingers had minor degenerative changes on radiographs [10].

Case Example

Dorsal block pinning is indicated for fractures >30 % of the articular surface of the volar base of the middle phalanx where congruent joint reduction can be obtained, but not maintained throughout the full arc of motion. In these patients, a dorsal, or extension, block pin can help to maintain the reduction while simultaneously allowing immediate motion within the stable arc to help prevent stiffness.

Case Example: A 44-year-old right-hand-dominant male injured his right small finger while playing broomball when the finger was hit by another player's stick. The patient noted immediate pain and deformity, but did not present for evaluation until 5 days after the injury. Radiographs obtained at that time demonstrated a dorsal fracture-dislocation of the PIPJ of the right small finger (Fig. 3.2). Because of the fracture pattern, as well as the time from injury to initial presentation, this was unable to be manipulated into a reduced position via closed methods in the clinic, and he was offered surgical intervention.

The patient was consented for possible closed versus open reduction and possible traction external fixation versus volar plate arthroplasty versus possible dorsal block pinning. He agreed to proceed as indicated at time of surgery. The patient was brought to the operating room and placed supine. He underwent induction of monitored anesthesia care. After appropriate prepping and draping, a digital block

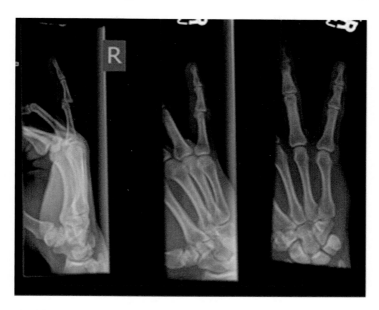

Fig. 3.2 Preoperative PA (**a**) and lateral (**b**) views of the small finger demonstrate a PIPJ fracture-dislocation with dorsal displacement of the middle phalanx

was performed with 10 ml of 1 % lidocaine 1:200,000 with epinephrine. After adequate anesthesia was achieved, the finger could be manipulated into a reduced position using a combination of traction and flexion at the PIP joint. The joint surface was congruent after reduction, however, was found to be exceedingly unstable and re-dislocated easily when the finger was extended. Due to the ability to obtain but not maintain a congruent joint reduction, decision was made to proceed with dorsal block pinning. A 0.054 in. K-wire was utilized as a dorsal blocking pin. This was placed in a percutaneous fashion through the distal head of the proximal phalanx and extending up the intramedullary canal. The wire was inserted in a slightly eccentric fashion to avoid the extensor apparatus dorsally and was placed in such a way as to hold the finger in approximately 10–15° more

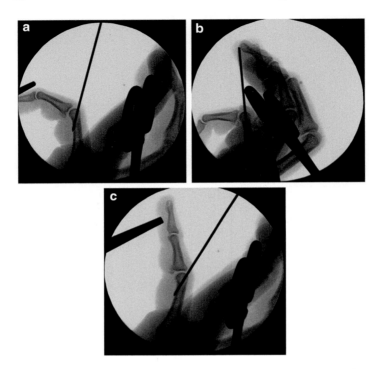

Fig. 3.3 Intraoperative fluoroscopic imaging demonstrating congruent reduction after placement of the K-wire (**a**). Note that reduction is maintained in full flexion (**b**) and maximal extension (**c**). With the K-wire in place, the joint lacks approximately 30° to full extension

flexion than the degree at which it re-dislocated (generally the pin will hold the PIPJ in about 30–40° of flexion (Fig. 3.3)).

The joint was then brought through a range of motion under fluoroscopy to verify that a congruent reduction was maintained throughout the arc of motion allowed by the presence of the dorsal K-wire. The K-wire was trimmed to length and left outside the skin. The patient was placed in a dorsal blocking alumifoam splint in the operating room after application of sterile dressings.

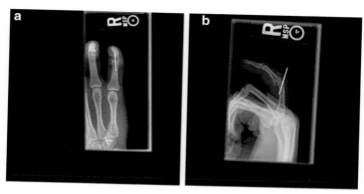

Fig. 3.4 PA (**a**) and lateral (**b**) radiographs obtained 3 weeks postoperatively demonstrate maintenance of a congruent joint reduction. The pin was subsequently removed

Supervised hand therapy was initiated on postoperative day 2 to allow full active flexion and extension as limited by the K-wire. A custom thermoplastic dorsal blocking splint was fabricated to protect the wire and for comfort. The patient worked closely with a hand therapist in order to ensure range of motion in the flexion arc was recovered. The patient was seen at approximately 3 weeks postoperatively and radiographs (Fig. 3.4) demonstrated maintenance of reduction. The K-wire was removed in the office and the patient continued to work in a supervised fashion to recover range of motion. The patient was last seen for follow-up on the day that the pin was removed. His ROM at the MP joint was 10–80° of flexion, PIP joint 30–80, and DIP joint 20–50. The patient was asked to follow-up in 2 weeks post-pin removal but declined to do so.

Summary

Proximal interphalangeal joint fracture-dislocations are common injuries and can lead to stiffness, pain, arthritis, and disability for patients. Fractures of the volar base of the middle phalanx that involve greater than 30 % of the articular surface are generally unstable after closed reduction and warrant operative treatment. Many methods have been described. Dorsal block pinning with a single K-wire is a satisfactory method to help hold the unstable joint congruently reduced during fracture healing. This avoids the need for cumbersome splinting and has the advantage of allowing immediate active motion of the finger within the confines of the wire and is minimally traumatic to the soft tissues.

References

1. Ng CY, Oliver CW. Fractures of the proximal interphalangeal joints of the fingers. J Bone Joint Surg Br. 2009;91(6):705–12. doi:10.1302/0301-620X.91B6.21953.
2. Badia A, Riano F, Ravikoff J, Khouri R, Gonzalez-Hernandez E, Orbay JL. Dynamic intradigital external fixation for proximal interphalangeal joint fracture dislocations. J Hand Surg Am. 2005;30(1):154–60. S0363-5023(04)00559-3 [pii].
3. Chinchalkar SJ, Gan BS. Management of proximal interphalangeal joint fractures and dislocations. J Hand Ther. 2003;16(2):117–28. S0894113003000255 [pii].
4. O'Rourke SK, Gaur S, Barton NJ. Long-term outcome of articular fractures of the phalanges: an eleven year follow up. J Hand Surg Br. 1989;14(2):183–93.
5. Vitale MA, White NJ, Strauch RJ. A percutaneous technique to treat unstable dorsal fracture-dislocations of the proximal interphalangeal joint. J Hand Surg Am. 2011;36(9):1453–9. doi:10.1016/j.jhsa.2011.06.022.
6. McElfresh EC, Dobyns JH, O'Brien ET. Management of fracture-dislocation of the proximal interphalangeal joints by extension-block splinting. J Bone Joint Surg Am. 1972;54(8):1705–11.
7. Sugawa I, Otani K, Kobayashi A. Treatment of fracture dislocation PIP-joint by kirschner wire extension block method. Cent Jpn J Orthop Traumat. 1979;22:1409–12.
8. Twyman RS, David HG. The doorstop procedure. A technique for treating unstable fracture dislocations of the proximal interphalangeal joint. J Hand Surg Br. 1993;18(6):714–5.
9. Viegas SF. Extension block pinning for proximal interphalangeal joint fracture dislocations: preliminary report of a new technique. J Hand Surg Am. 1992;17(5):896–901.
10. Waris E, Alanen V. Percutaneous, intramedullary fracture reduction and extension block pinning for dorsal proximal interphalangeal fracture-dislo-

cations. J Hand Surg Am. 2010;35(12):2046–52. doi:10.1016/j.jhsa.2010.08.004.

11. Inoue G, Tamura Y. Treatment of fracture-dislocation of the proximal interphalangeal joint using extension-block kirschner wire. Ann Chir Main Memb Super. 1991;10(6):564–8.

Chapter 4
Proximal Interphalangeal Joint Fracture-Dislocations: Closed Reduction Internal Fixation

Mark A. Vitale and Robert J. Strauch

Abstract This chapter will review closed reduction internal fixation (CRIF) of proximal interphalangeal (PIP) joint fracture-dislocations, including transarticular pinning, extension block pinning, and various techniques of closed reduction and percutaneous pinning (CRPP). While the vast majority of dislocations are dorsal, we will also briefly discuss CRIF of PIP joint palmar fracture-dislocations, a less commonly encountered pattern of injury.

Keywords Proximal interphalangeal (PIP) joint • Closed reduction and internal fixation (CRIF) • Transarticular pinning • Extension block pinning • Closed reduction and percutaneous pinning (CRPP)

M.A. Vitale, M.D., M.P.H.
ONS Foundation, 6 Greenwich Office Park, 40 Valley Drive,
Greenwich, CT 06831, USA
e-mail: markavitale@yahoo.com

R.J. Strauch, M.D. (✉)
Department of Orthopaedic Surgery, New York-Presbyterian Medical Center,
Columbia University, 622 West 168th Street, PH 1119, 11th Floor,
New York, NY 10032, USA
e-mail: robertjstrauch@hotmail.com

© Springer International Publishing Switzerland 2016   43
J.E. Adams (ed.), *PIP Joint Fracture Dislocations*,
DOI 10.1007/978-3-319-28579-5_4

PIP Joint Dorsal Fracture-Dislocations

Introduction

PIP joint dorsal fracture-dislocations are injuries that occur most commonly as the result of an axial force to a hyperextended finger, and they represent a wide spectrum of injuries [1]. Currently no one surgical procedure has proven superiority in achieving the goal of achieving and maintaining a concentric joint reduction in the setting of the unstable PIP fracture-dislocation (those fracture-dislocations in which the volar fragment represents >40 % of the joint surface) [3–6]. Numerous different techniques have been described, reflecting the lack of consensus [1, 7–9]. This section will review methods of acute treatment of PIP joint dorsal fracture-dislocations with closed reduction and internal fixation (CRIF), including transarticular pinning, and numerous methods of closed reduction and percutaneous pinning (CRPP). The benefit of using methods of CRIF to treat dorsal fracture-dislocations is avoidance of an open approach to the joint which may promote scarring of the joint capsule and tendons, but truly anatomic reduction of the fracture fragments may not be possible with these techniques. It has been reported that reduction of joint subluxation and not anatomic reduction of articular fragments is the most important determinant of outcome, thereby making CRPP an attractive option [7, 8]. The treatment of chronic PIP fracture-dislocations will not be discussed in this chapter.

Transarticular Pinning

The technique of transarticular pinning for unstable dorsal PIP fracture-dislocations dates back to descriptions by Bunnell [10] and later Boyes [11], Spray [12], Milford [13], and Barton [14]. Bunnell's initial technique involved manual closed reduction of the fracture-dislocation followed by a transarticular wire inserted dorsally into the middle phalanx through the PIP joint and into the proximal phalanx. Barton later elaborated that the K-wire should be introduced distal to the insertion of the central slip and proximal to the conjunction of the lateral slips and removed 3–4 weeks later.

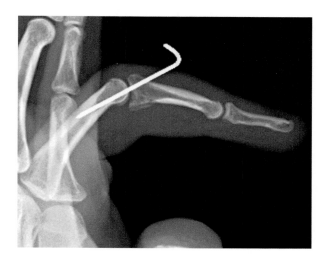

Fig. 4.1 Transarticular wire to hold reduction of dorsal PIP fracture-dislocation. (With permission from de Haseth, K.B., Neuhaus, V. and Mugdal, C.S.
Dorsal fracture-dislocations of the proximal interphalangeal joint: evaluation
of closed reduction and percutaneous Kirschner wire pinning. HAND 2015.
10:88–93)

Newington, Davis, and Barton described their technique in a series
of ten patients (Fig. 4.1) [15]. The authors performed a closed
reduction of the unstable dorsal fracture-dislocation and then stabilized the PIP joint in 20–40° of flexion with a transarticular K-wire
which was left in place for 3 weeks. At a mean of 16 years of
follow-up, they reported a mean ROM of the PIP joint of 85°.
While the use of a percutaneously placed transarticular wire holds
the joint reduced in the postoperative period, the disadvantage is
that no motion may be initiated while the K-wire is in place.

Haseth, Neuhaus, and Mudgal recently reported the results of nine
patients treated with closed reduction and transarticular pinning [16].
K-wires were removed at an average of 28 days. At a mean follow-up
of 6.5 months, the average PIP joint motion was 106° of flexion and
4° short of full extension, and no patients reported pain at final
follow-up. Two patients had radiographic evidence of degenerative
changes at the PIP joint but were asymptomatic, and one patient
developed a transient superficial pin track infection, K-wire breakage,
mild subluxation of the PIP joint, and avascular necrosis of one of the
condyles of the proximal phalanx at 20-month follow-up.

Closed Reduction and Percutaneous Pinning

Different methods using percutaneously placed K-wires for reduction and/or fixation of the displaced volar fracture fragments have been described with success. Lahav, Teplitz, and McCormack described a technique utilizing CRPP to treat either fractures of the volar lip of the middle phalanx without an associated dislocation or impacted intra-articular fractures of the middle phalanx in five patients [19]. They describe using a 0.035″ K-wire placed through the dorsal cortex of the middle phalanx to manipulate impacted articular fragments, followed by insertion of four 0.028″ K-wires for fixation of the fracture fragments (two volar-dorsal and two radial-ulnar). These authors reported an average ROM at the PIP joint from −1° to 95° and 4–68° at the DIP joint, but it should be noted that this technique was designed to treat PIP fractures without dislocation and impaction fractures, not PIP fracture-dislocations.

Waris and Alanen described a method of percutaneous fracture reduction and dorsal block pinning in 15 dorsal PIP fracture-dislocations [20]. This technique involves first performing a closed reduction and dorsal block pinning. A pre-bent 1.0-mm K-wire is then inserted percutaneously through a 2.0-mm cortical hole in the distal aspect of the middle phalanx and passed through the intramedullary canal of the middle phalanx from a distal to proximal direction to disimpact and reduce the volar articular fragments of the PIP joint under fluoroscopic guidance (Fig. 4.2a–e). This wire is removed intraoperatively, leaving only the dorsal blocking wire in place. The authors recommended passive ROM exercises at the PIP joint started initially within the limits of the extension blocking K-wire, with active ROM of the metacarpophalangeal (MCP) and DIP joints begun immediately postoperatively. After 2–4 weeks the dorsal blocking wire is removed and therapy is started with free passive and active mobilization of the joint. At 5-year follow-up, reduction of the joint was maintained, articular step-off was reduced, and PIP motion averaged 83°, with a mean flexion contracture of 3°.

Vitale, White, and Strauch described a technique referred to as closed reduction dorsal block pinning and percutaneous reduction

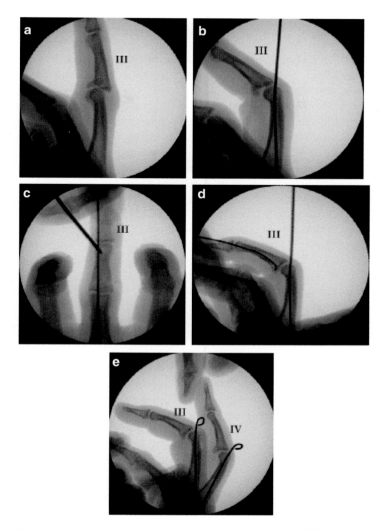

Fig. 4.2 Lateral fluoroscopic view (a) of middle finger of dorsal PIP joint fracture-dislocation. After inserting extension block pinning (b), the joint is concentrically reduced, but fracture fragments remain displaced. A 2.0-mm cortical hole is made percutaneously in the distal aspect of middle phalanx (c), and a pre-bent 1.0-mm K-wire is inserted through this cortical window and the medullary cavity in the middle phalanx down to the fracture site to disimpact the articular fragments (d). Final appearance revealing articular congruency of middle finger and similarly treated ring finger injury (e) following removal of the intramedullary K-wire. (With permission from E Waris and V Alanen. Percutaneous, intramedullary fracture reduction and extension block pinning for dorsal proximal interphalangeal fracture-dislocations. J Hand Surg 2010;35A:2046–2052)

(CRDBPPR) that utilizes a combination of volar- to dorsal-directed percutaneous pinning of the volar fracture fragments and dorsal block pinning in a series of six patients with unstable dorsal fracture-dislocations of the PIP joint [21]. In their series at an average follow-up of 17 months, there were no postoperative episodes of subluxation or dislocation, the mean range of motion was 4° of extension to 93° of flexion at the PIP joint and 1° of extension to 73° of flexion at the DIP joint, and radiographic data confirmed concentric reduction with patient-based measures indicating high levels of function and little or no pain.

A typical patient treated with the CRDCPPR technique by the senior author is presented. This patient was a 29-year-old male who injured his right middle finger playing football. Preoperative radiographs revealed a dorsally displaced PIP joint fracture-dislocation with the volar fragment comprising about 45 % of the articular surface (Fig. 4.3a, b). In the operating room, an attempt was made to perform a closed reduction, but intraoperative fluoroscopy revealed persistent subluxation. The uninvolved fingers were wrapped with gauze in order to flex the unaffected digits into the palm, leaving only the injured digit free (Fig. 4.4a). The fluoroscopy machine was brought into the field in the horizontal position for ease of K-wire placement and visualization. A large pointed towel clip was used for reduction of the volar fragment to the intact dorsal base with one point placed percutaneously onto the mid-dorsal base of the proximal phalanx and the other point inserted through the skin directly into the volar fragment through the midline of the flexor tendons (Fig. 4.4b). Extremely gentle compression was applied in order to reduce the volar fragment to the dorsal intact middle phalangeal base with percutaneous manipulation of the palmar fragment using the towel clip. This is performed with the patient's hand in the supinated position such that a true magnified lateral image can be easily viewed. Once an adequate reduction was seen on fluoroscopy, a 0.028 K-wire was inserted by hand immediately lateral to either side of the volar limb of the towel clip under fluoroscopy just distal to the articular surface (Fig. 4.4c). The K-wires therefore passed through the flexor tendons in the area of the PIP joint, and, if the towel clip is positioned directly midline, the neurovascular bundles are not at risk of injury.

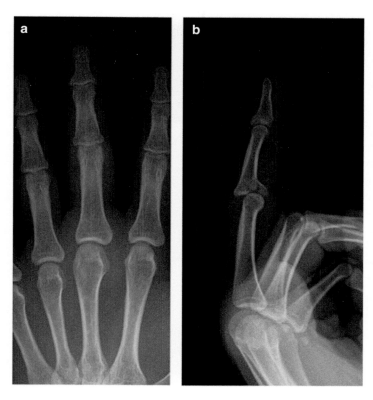

Fig. 4.3 Preoperative posteroanterior (a) and lateral (b) radiographs of a dorsal PIP joint fracture-dislocation with involvement of approximately 40–50 % of the joint surface and significant dorsal subluxation. (Radiographs with permission from RJ Strauch)

The 0.028 K-wires were then driven under power across the dorsal middle phalangeal cortex and out the dorsal skin. They were retrieved from the dorsal side of the finger and withdrawn until they are seen to be nearly level with the volar aspect of the volar fracture fragment. In order to ensure that the PIP joint remains located in the postoperative period, a "blocking" 0.035 K-wire was then skived along the dorsal rim of the middle phalanx base in the midline to engage the head of the proximal phalanx (Fig. 4.4d).

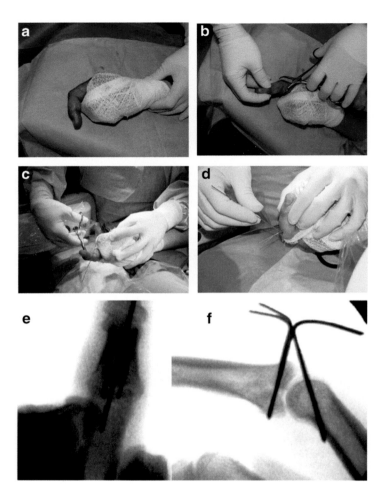

Fig. 4.4 Preoperative position of the hand on a mini c-arm for a percutaneous closed reduction allows a lateral fluoroscopic view of the reduction, with the uninvolved fingers wrapped in a gauze wrap (a). A large pointed towel clamp is utilized for a very gentle reduction of fracture with the clamp ends inserted onto the dorsal base of the proximal phalanx and the volar fragment through the midline of the flexor tendon percutaneously (b). Two 0.028 K-wires are inserted immediately lateral to either side of the volar end of the clamp under fluoroscopic visualization, placing the wires just distal to the articular surface (c). A 0.035 blocking K-wire is then inserted along the dorsal rim of the middle phanalgeal base in the midline of the coronal plane into the head of the proximal phalanx to keep the middle phalanx reduced (d). Posteroanterior (e) and lateral (f) intraoperative fluoroscopic views after reduction, percutaneous K-wire fixation and dorsal blocking K-wire. (Clinical photos and radiographs with permission from RJ Strauch)

The K-wires were bent 90° to prevent retraction under the skin, and final fluoroscopic images verified the reduction (Fig. 4.4e, f). Volar and dorsal splints from the distal forearm to but not including the dorsal interphalangeal (DIP) joint level were applied, incorporating the affected finger and an adjacent digit.

The patient was kept in the operative splint until the first postoperative visit at approximately 10–14 days; DIP but not PIP motion was allowed while in the splint. The pin sites were cleaned with alcohol and new splints are applied. At 4 weeks time, the K-wires were removed after radiographic verification of maintenance of reduction (Fig. 4.5a, b). When the pins were removed, active and forceful flexor tendon contraction is performed to rupture the developing flexor adhesions. This is performed by providing a digital block with a combination of 1 % lidocaine and 0.25 % marcaine. With the PIP joint held in a stable position with one thumb gently keeping the dorsal middle phalangeal base in place, the DIP joint is passively manipulated into full extension or hyperextension, at which time some adhesions will usually be felt to tear free. The patient is then asked to maximally make a fist with all fingers and rupture of remaining flexor tendon adhesions may be palpated. Typically, PIP flexion to 90° is possible after several minutes, though the DIP joint is usually unable to fully flex due to stiffness. The patient was then placed into a dorsal blocking AlumaFoam splint secured to the dorsal proximal phalanx with tape and blocking PIP extension at 20°. Full active flexion and extension within the confines of the splint are begun immediately and hand therapy is initiated. A week later, radiographs were checked to verify maintenance of reduction, and full use without splinting is allowed by 6–8 weeks when final radiographs are obtained to verify maintenance of reduction and union of the fracture (Fig. 4.5c, d).

Most reported series of PIP fracture-dislocations make no mention of DIP range of motion of the injured finger. Despite direct injury to the PIP joint (without injury to DIP), it is quite common to also develop DIP joint stiffness during treatment; this DIP stiffness may be permanent [7]. DIP stiffness may result from finger swelling, collateral ligament and capsular contracture, extensor tendon adhesions, or lack of focus on DIP rehabilitation. Whatever the reason, a patient with an excellent PIP joint ROM of 0–95° may still be dissatisfied if

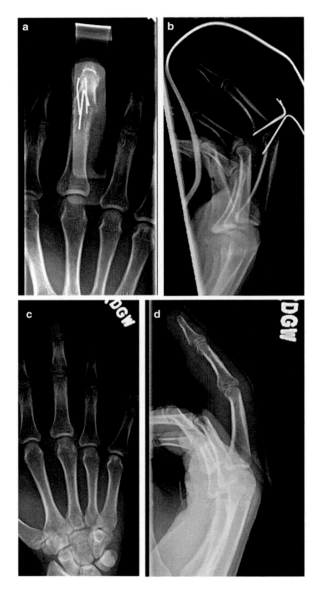

Fig. 4.5 Postoperative posteroanterior (a) and lateral (b) radiographs obtained at 4 weeks postop just prior to pin removal. Posterioanterior (a) and lateral (b) radiographs obtained at 6 weeks postop verifying maintenance of reduction and progression of fracture union. (Radiographs with permission from RJ Strauch)

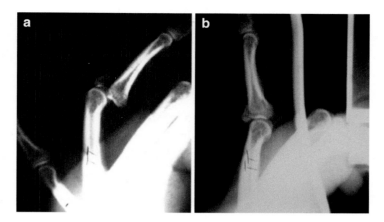

Fig. 4.6 Laterral prereduction radiograph (a) of a palmar PIP joint fracture-dislocation. Postreduction radiograph (b) reveals relovation of the PIP joint and reduction of the fracture fragment. (With permission from RP Calfee and TG Sommerkamp. Fracture-dislocation about the finger joints. J Hand Surg 2009;34A:1140–1147)

the DIP joint flexes only 10°, leading to inability to make a tight fist and the fingertip remaining extended when making a fist. Therefore, careful attention should be paid towards regaining not only PIP but also DIP motion during rehabilitation of these injuries.

PIP Joint Palmar Fracture-Dislocations

Palmar fracture-dislocations represent a much less frequently encountered pattern of injury. The mechanism of injury is thought to be an axial load with a palmar-directed force over the middle phalangeal base [22]. Rosenstadt et al. reported on treatment of 13 patients with palmar fracture-dislocation of the PIP joint, nine of which were acute injuries and four of which were chronic (treated more than 1 month after injury) [23]. The authors reported that reducing the joint dislocation or subluxation without fixation of the fracture fragments was frequently sufficient to reduce the associated dorsal middle phalangeal base fracture (Fig. 4.6a, b). Of the acute injuries in their series, seven of nine were treated with CRPP

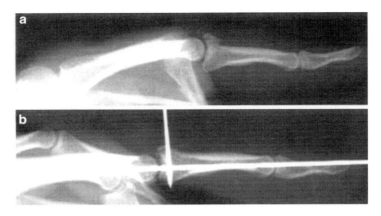

Fig. 4.7 Palmar fracture-dislocation with comminuted dorsal fragment as viewed on lateral radiograph (a) treated with closed reduction and percutaneous pinning with a transarticular K-wire (b). (With permission from BE Rosenstadt, et al. Palmar fracture dislocation of the proximal interphalangeal joint. J Hand Surg 1998;23A:811–820)

(Fig. 4.7a, b) and two were treated with ORIF, whereas all chronic injuries were treated with open reduction and soft tissue reconstruction. At an average of 55-month follow-up, PIP motion averaged 91° for acute injuries and 71° for chronic injuries, and overall 8 of 13 patients were pain-free. Radiographic abnormalities including increased posteroanterior height of the base of the middle phalanx, articular irregularity, and subluxation were common, but these findings did not correlate with clinical results. Complications included loss of reduction in one patient, a progressive swan neck deformity in 1, and a 25° average DIP lag in 5 of 13 patients.

Summary/Conclusions

For PIP joint dorsal fracture-dislocations, it remains unclear what method of surgical stabilization results in the optimal outcome [7–9], and to date there are no prospective randomized trials comparing different methods of treatment for these injuries.

For unstable injuries dorsal extension block or transarticular pinning will better control the tendency for dorsal subluxation/ dislocation than dorsal block splinting and has been shown to yield long-term satisfactory results. Various methods of CRPP (in addition to transarticular or dorsal block pinning) may be especially useful to better reduce displaced volar fragments, although achieving a concentric reduction seems to be more important than anatomic reduction of the articular surface [7, 8]. Maintaining functional motion at the DIP joint is also of paramount importance.

References

1. Ng CY, Oliver CW. Fractures of the proximal interphalangeal joints of the fingers. J Bone Joint Surg Br. 2009;91-B:705–12.
2. O'Rourke SK, Gauer S, Barton NJ. Long-term outcome of articular fractures of the phalanges: an eleven year follow-up. J Hand Surg Br. 1989; 14:183–93.
3. McElfresh EC, Dobyns JH, O'Brien ET. Management of fracture-dislocation of the proximal interphalangeal joints by extension-block splinting. J Bone Joint Surg Am. 1972;54-A:1705–11.
4. Strong ML. A new method of extension-block splinting for the proximal interphalangeal joint: preliminary report. J Hand Surg Am. 1980;5: 606–7.
5. Williams CS. Proximal interphalangeal joint fracture dislocations: stable and unstable. Hand Clin. 2012;28:409–16.
6. Kiefhaber TR, Stern PJ. Fracture dislocations of the proximal interphalangeal joint. J Hand Surg Am. 1998;23A:368–80.
7. Deitch MA, Kiefhaber TR, Comisar BR, Stern PJ. Dorsal fracture dislocations of the proximal interphalangeal joint: surgical complications and long-term results. J Hand Surg Am. 1999;24:914–23.
8. Aladin A, Davis TRC. Dorsal fracture-dislocation of the proximal interphalangeal joint: a comparative study of percutaneous Kirschner wire fixation versus open reduction and internal fixation. J Hand Surg Br. 2005;30B:120–8.
9. Barksfield RC, Bowden B, Chojnowski AJ. Hemi-hamate arthroplasty versus transarticular Kirschner wire fixation for unstable dorsal fracture-dislocation of the proximal interphalangeal joint in the hand. Hand Surg. 2015;20:115–9.
10. Bunnell S. Surgery of the hand. 3rd ed. Philadelphia, PA: JB Lippincott; 1956.
11. Boyes JH. Bunnell's surgery of the hand. 4th ed. Philadelphia, PA: JB Lippincott; 1964. p. 650–7.

12. Spray P. Finger fracture-dislocation proximal at the interphalangeal joint. J Tenn Med Assoc. 1966;59:765–6.
13. Milford L. The hand. In: Campbell's operative orthopaedics. 5th ed. St Louis, MO: CV Mosby; 1971. p. 199–200.
14. Barton NJ. Fractures of the hand. J Bone Joint Surg Br. 1984;66-B: 159–67.
15. Newington DP, Davis TRC, Barton NJ. The treatment of dorsal fracture-dislocation of the proximal interphalangeal joint by closed reduction and Kirschner wire fixation: a 16-year follow up. J Hand Surg Br. 2001; 26-B(6):537–40.
16. de Haseth KB, Neuhaus V, Mudgal CS. Dorsal fracture-dislocations of the proximal interphalangeal joint: evaluation of closed reduction and percutaneous Kirschner wire pinning. Hand (N Y). 2015;10:88–93.
16. Sugawa I, Otani K, Kobayashi A. Treatment of fracture dislocation PIP-joint by Kirschner wire extension block method. Cent Jpn J Orthop Traumat. 1979;22:1409–12.
17. Viegas SF. Extension block pinning for proximal interphalangeal joint fracture dislocations: preliminary report of a new technique. J Hand Surg Am. 1992;17A:896–901.
18. Twyman RS, David HG. The doorstop procedure. J Hand Surg Br. 1993; 18B:714–5.
19. Inoue G, Tamura Y. Treatment of fracture-dislocation of the proximal interphalangeal joint using extension-block Kirschner wire. Ann Chir Main Mem Super. 1991;10:564–8.
20. Lahav A, Teplitz GA, McCormack Jr RR. Percutaneous reduction and Kirschner-wire fixation of impacted intra-articular fractures and volar lip fractures of the proximal interphalangeal joint. Am J Orthop. 2005; 34:62–5.
21. Waris E, Alanen A. Percutaneous, intramedullary fracture reduction and extension block pinning for dorsal proximal interphalangeal fracture-dislocations. J Hand Surg Am. 2010;35A:2046–52.
22. Vitale MA, White NJ, Strauch RJ. A percutaneous technique to treat unstable dorsal fracture-dislocation of the proximal interphalangeal joint. J Hand Surg Am. 2011;36A:1453–9.
23. Calfee RP, Sommerkamp MD. Fracture-dislocations about the finger joints. J Hand Surg Am. 2009;34A:1140–7.
24. Rosenstadt BE, Glickel SZ, Lane LB, Kaplan SJ. Palmar fracture dislocation of the proximal interphalangeal joint. J Hand Surg Am. 1998; 23A:811–20.

Chapter 5
External Fixation of PIP Joint Dorsal Fracture-Dislocations

Stephanie Sweet and Lawrence E. Weiss

Abstract Dorsal PIP joint fracture-dislocations are challenging injuries. Dynamic external fixation devices are ideal to restore congruency and stability and to allow for early controlled motion, particularly in the settings of dorsal fracture-dislocations, pilon fractures, and selected complex middle phalanx fractures. This technique may be used as an adjunctive treatment to open or percutaneous fixation. Contraindications include chronic injury, certain fractures involving P1 or P2 head/neck, poor skin coverage, and significant preexisting arthritis. Dynamic wire-form traction with rubber band technique (Suzuki) and without rubber band technique (push traction) are both illustrated. Reverse push traction is also demonstrated. The authors demonstrate the tips and techniques and pearls of application of traction/external fixation.

S. Sweet, M.D. (✉)
Philadelphia Hand Center, Thomas Jefferson University,
700 S. Henderson Road, King of Prussia, PA 19406, USA
e-mail: ssweet@handcenters.com

L.E. Weiss, M.D.
Division of Hand Surgery, OAA Hand Center, Lehigh Valley Hospital,
250 Cetronia Road, Second Floor, Allentown, PA 18104, USA
e-mail: lweiss@oaainstitute.com

© Springer International Publishing Switzerland 2016   57
J.E. Adams (ed.), *PIP Joint Fracture Dislocations*,
DOI 10.1007/978-3-319-28579-5_5

Keywords   PIP joint fracture-dislocation • Suzuki • Push traction • External fixation for PIP joint • Dynamic traction • Pilon fracture PIP joint

Important Concepts in Treatment of PIP Injuries

- Dynamic external fixator works through ligamentotaxis.
- Goal of any treatment is to restore a stable and congruent joint.
- Any type of treatment should allow initiation of early ROM.
- Nonanatomic articular alignment may be acceptable.
- Radiographic arthritis posttreatment may not necessarily be symptomatic.

Indications for PIP External Fixator

- Dorsal fracture-dislocations
- Pilon fractures of the P2 base
- Selected comminuted, complex middle phalanx shaft/base fractures
- Adjunctive treatment to other percutaneous or open approaches

Contraindications to Wire-Form Dynamic PIP Fixator

- Chronic injury
- Segmental digital injuries compromising the P1 or P2 head
- Significant preexisting arthritis
- Simultaneous need for reconstructive soft-tissue coverage

Case Presentation

Twenty-nine-year-old right-hand-dominant male sustained an axial load to his right ring finger. Physical exam revealed pain and swelling at the PIP joint. Range of motion was 20–40° at the PIP joint. The flexor tendons were intact and the neurovascular status was normal. Radiographs revealed an unstable dorsal PIP joint fracture-dislocation (shown below).

Push traction was utilized to restore PIP congruity and enable early recovery of range of motion.

Dynamic Wire-Form Rubber Band Traction

- Popularized by Suzuki (later Slade).
- Middle phalanx is distracted using rubber band system.

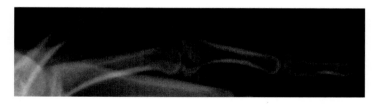

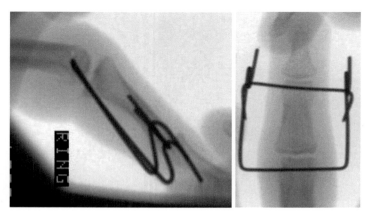

- Pins placed in the center of the P1 and P2 heads and middle of the P2 base.
- Blocking pin in the middle phalanx allows for volar PIP translation.
- Advantages: inexpensive, reasonable outcomes compared to open treatment.
- Disadvantages: bulky, rubber band breakage, pin tract issues, and learning curve.

Dynamic Wire-Form Traction Without Rubber Bands (Push Traction)

- Popularized by Gaul.
- Middle phalanx is distracted through wire tension.
- Pins placed in the center of the P1 and P2 heads (only).
- No blocking pin, so no volarly directed translation force (straight distraction only).
- Advantages: inexpensive, no rubber band breakage, similar outcomes to Suzuki.
- Disadvantages: no blocking pin, pin tract issues.

Suzuki Rubber Band Traction

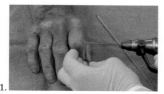

1.
0.045 K-wire placed in center of P1 head

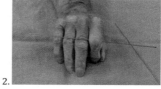

2.
Pin advanced across P1 head

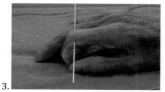

3.
Side view of advanced pin

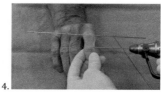

4.
0.045 K wire placed in center of P2 head

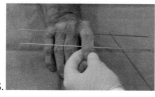

5.
Pin advanced across P2 head

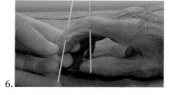

6.
Side view of advanced pin

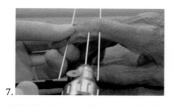

7.
0.045 K-wire placed in center of P2 base

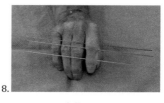

8.
Front view of all 3 pins in position

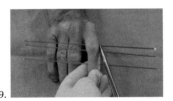

9.

Needle driver placed on
proximal wire near skin

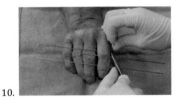

10.

Bend pin 90°

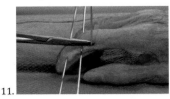

11.

Side view of proximal pin bend

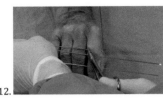

12.

Perform similar bend on opposite side

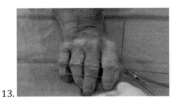

13.

Configuration of pins after bending

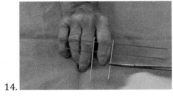

14.

Needle driver grab wire 1 cm
distal to the fingertip

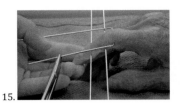

15.

Side view of distal pin grab

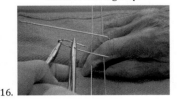

16.

Bend tip of pin proximally over
needle driver

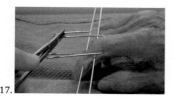

17.

Grab dorsal limb 1 cm from distal bend

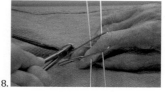

18.

Bend tip of pin distally over
needle driver

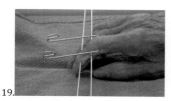

19.

Distal horns created after cutting excess

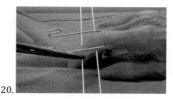

20.

Needle driver placed on
distal wire near skin

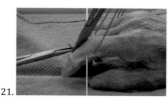

21.

Distal wires bent and cut into hooks

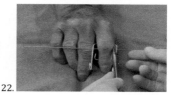

22.

Proximal P2 pin bent around P1 pin

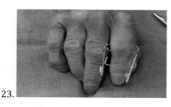

23.

Construct with proximal P2 pin bent

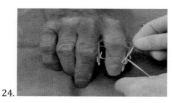

24.

Vessel loop secures traction
between distal horn and P2 hooks

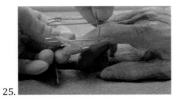

25.

Side view of vessel loop application

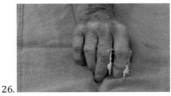

26.

Final construct Suzuki
rubberband traction

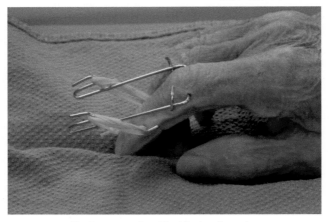

Final construct Suzuki rubberband traction

Push Traction

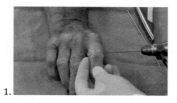

1.

0.045 K-wire placed in center of P1 head

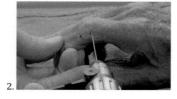

2.

Side view of P1 pin

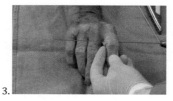

3.

Pin advanced across P1 head

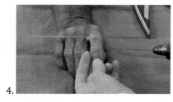

4.

0.045 K wire placed in center of
P2 head

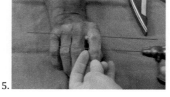

5.

Pin advanced across P2 head

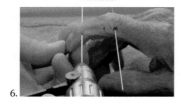

6.

Side view of advanced pin

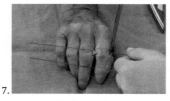

7.

Needle driver placed on
proximal wire near skin

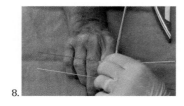

8.

Bend pin 90°

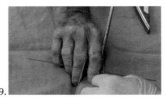

9.

Configuration of pins after bending

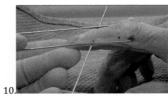

10.

Side view after P1 pin bends

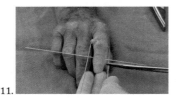

11.

Needle driver grab wire 1 cm
distal to the P2 wire

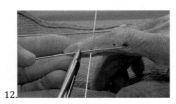

12.

Side view of P1 wire distal pin
grab

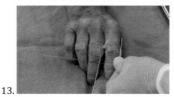

13.

Bend tip of pin proximally over
needle driver

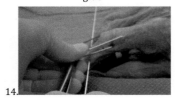

14.

Side view of proximal bend of P1 wire

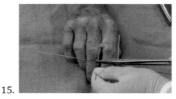

15.

Bend opposite side of
construct in similar fashion

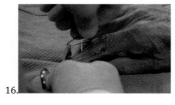

16.

Side view of opposite side bend

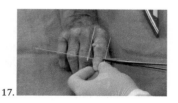

Grab dorsal limb 1-2 mm distal to P2 pin

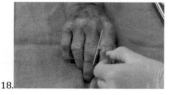

Bend tip of pin distally over
needle driver

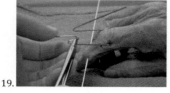

Side view of distal limb bend

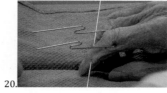

Side view of distal horns

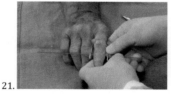

Engage P2 pin into P1 horns

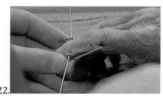

Side view of P2 pin engaged into
P1 horns

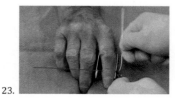

Grab P2 pin at skin to bend around horns

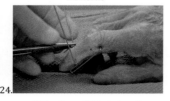

Side view of P2 pin bends
around P1 horns

25.

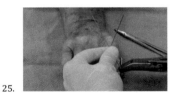

Cut excess P2 pin

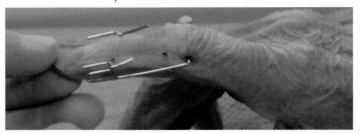

Final construct push traction

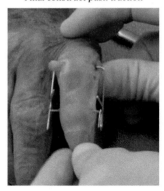

Final construct push traction

Reverse Push Traction

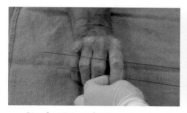

Similar P1 and P2 center head
0.045 K-wires

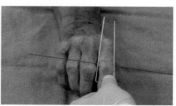

Instead of using P1 pin bent
distal, P2 pin is bent proximal

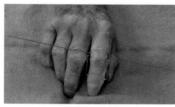

P2 pin engages P1 pin proximally

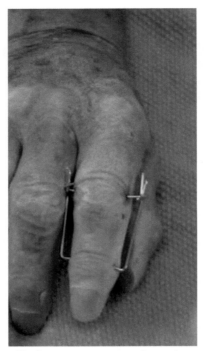

Final construct reverse push traction

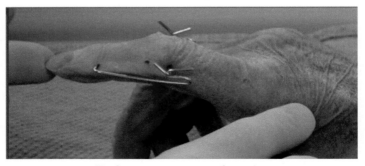

Final construct reverse push traction

Pearls for PIP External Fixator Application

- Initially place pins unicortical and check on c-arm to avoid over-perforating (and weakening) the far cortex. This also allows fine-tuning on the AP view.
- If the pin is not at first perfectly in the center of the proximal/middle phalanx head, leave pin in (cut it short) and use its location as a reference for a second attempt.
- The mid-axis of the phalanx skeleton is more dorsal than you think based on its surface anatomy.
- Overbend the P1 proximal pin at PIP level bend to achieve a parallel pin alignment with the longitudinal axis of the finger (gives better vector of distraction).
- C-wires may be used instead of K-wires in push traction applications, as the pins don't need to be as long (easier to c-arm with C-wires). K-wires are mandatory in Suzuki traction (at least for the P1 pin).
- Cover the cut pin ends with Coban or Steri-Strips to avoid the sharp edges.

Postoperative Management

Postoperatively, patients are seen within a few days by the surgeon and hand therapist to start a supervised exercise program. It is wise to have the patient followed closely to insure that the wires do not become bent or the rubber bands do not come off or break and to monitor for pin track issues. The patient is allowed to move within the confines of the fixator device and encouraged to work on arc of motion. The fixator device is typically removed between 3 and 6 weeks postoperatively. In the setting of rubber band devices, it is often helpful to remove the rubber bands and then obtain a fluoroscopic view of the digit as the finger is flexed and extended, to ensure that motion remains congruent and the joint remains reduced. If this is the case, the fixator device is cut and removed. Patients continue a supervised therapy program to regain motion.

Suggested Readings

1. Inanami H, Ninomiya S, Okutsu I, Tarui T. Dynamic external finger fixator for fracture dislocation of the proximal interphalangeal joint. J Hand Surg Am. 1993;18A:160–4.
2. Suzuki Y, Matsunaga T, Sato S, Yokoi T. The pins and rubber traction system for treatment of comminuted intra-articular fractures and fracture dislocations in the hand. J Hand Surg Br. 1994;19B:98–107.
3. DeSoras X, DeMourgues P, Guinard D, Moutet F. Pins and rubbers traction system. J Hand Surg Br. 1997;22B:730–5.
4. Bain GI, Mehta JA, Heptinstall RJ, Bria M. Dynamic external fixation for injuries of the proximal interphalangeal joint. J Bone Joint Surg Br. 1998; 80:1014–9.
5. Gaul Jr JS, Rosenberg SN. Fracture-dislocation of the middle phalanx at the proximal interphalangeal joint: repair with a simple intradigital traction-fixation device. Am J Orthop. 1998;27:682–8.
6. DeSmet L, Fabry G. Treatment of fracture-dislocations of the proximal interphalangeal joint with the "pins & rubbers" traction system. Acta Ortho Belgica. 1998;64:229–32.
7. Hynes MC, Giddins GE. Dynamic external fixation for pilon fractures of the interphalangeal joints. J Hand Surg Br. 2001;26B:122–4.
8. Syed AA, Agarwal M, Boome R. Dynamic external fixator for pilon fractures of the proximal interphalangeal joints: a simple fixator for a complex fracture. J Hand Surg Br. 2003;28B:137–41.
9. Johnson D, Tiernan E, Richards AM, Cole RP. Dynamic external fixation for complex intraarticular phalangeal fractures. J Hand Surg Br. 2004;29B: 76–81.
10. Deshmukh SC, Kumar D, Mathur K, Thomas B. Complex fracture-dislocation of the proximal interphalangeal joint of the hand. Results of a modified pins and rubbers traction system. J Bone Joint Surg. 2004; 86B:406–12.
11. Badia A, Riano F, Ravikoff J, Khouri R, Orbay JL, Gonzalez-Hernandez E. Dynamic intradigital external fixation for proximal interphalangeal joint fracture dislocations. J Hand Surg Am. 2005;30A:154–60.
12. Ellis SJ, Cheng R, Prokopis P, Chetboun A, Wolfe SW, Athanasian EA, Weiland AJ. Treatment of proximal interphalangeal dorsal fracture-dislocation injuries with dynamic external fixation: a pins and rubber band system. J Hand Surg Am. 2007;32A:1242–50.
13. Ruland RT, Hogan CJ, Cannon DL, Slade JF. Use of dynamic distraction external fixation for unstable fracture-dislocations of the proximal interphalangeal joint. J Hand Surg Am. 2008;33A:19–25.

Chapter 6
Use of Force Couple Devices for Treatment of PIP Fracture-Dislocations

Maureen O'Shaughnessy and Marco Rizzo

Abstract   Successful management of proximal interphalangeal joint fracture-dislocations can be challenging. Patients with unstable joints and intact dorsal column may often be successfully treated with a force couple device. Its application can be performed percutaneously and allows for early range-of-motion while maintaining a congruent joint. This chapter illustrates a case example with management using a force couple device.

Keywords   Proximal interphalangeal joint • Fracture-dislocation • Force couple device

Case Presentation

A 51-year-old right hand-dominant male manual laborer presented with pain, deformity, and swelling over the proximal interphalangeal (PIP) joint of the right ring finger. The patient reported falling from a ground level height onto the hand with the right ring finger in a straightened posture, resulting in an axial load to the digit.

M. O'Shaughnessy, M.D. • M. Rizzo, M.D. (✉)
Department of Orthopedic Surgery, Mayo Clinic,
200 First St. SW, Rochester, MN 55905, USA
e-mail: Rizzo.marco@mayo.edu

© Springer International Publishing Switzerland 2016   73
J.E. Adams (ed.), *PIP Joint Fracture Dislocations*,
DOI 10.1007/978-3-319-28579-5_6

Physical Assessment

The physical exam demonstrated intact skin and essentially no motion at the PIP joint. Substantial swelling was appreciated over the digit. Stressing of the joint was limited secondary to pain. Neurovascular exam demonstrated two-point discrimination of 5 mm in the radial and ulnar digital nerve distributions concordant with his other digits. He also had less than 2 s capillary refill, similar to other digits.

Diagnostic Studies and Diagnosis

Anteroposterior (AP), oblique, and lateral radiographs (Fig. 6.1) demonstrated a comminuted ring finger middle phalanx fracture and subluxation of the PIP joint. Notably, the dorsal column of the base of the proximal phalanx remained intact. Overall alignment on the PA view was appropriate. His diagnosis was a right ring finger PIP fracture-dislocation.

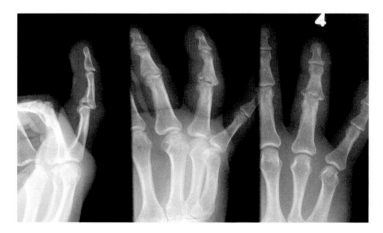

Fig. 6.1 PA, oblique, and lateral films of the right ring finger of a 51-year-old male who sustained a dorsal fracture-dislocation of the PIP joint. Note that the dorsal cortex of the middle phalanx is intact

Management Options

The key to successful treatment of these injuries lies in maintaining congruency of the joint. Both surgical and nonsurgical treatments can be utilized for PIP fracture-dislocations. Nonoperative interventions include extension block splinting. Surgical treatments include extension block pinning, PIP joint reduction and pinning, open reduction and internal fixation, static external fixation, and dynamic external fixation.

Management Chosen

Since this fracture was comminuted with a substantial portion of the base of the middle phalanx affected, closed reduction and splinting were unsuccessful in maintaining the joint congruency. Thus, extension block splinting did not appear to be a viable option. Open reduction and internal fixation was also thought likely to be unsuccessful due to the extensive comminution of the fracture. The surgical option selected for this injury was to create a dynamic external fixation device or force couple device that could maintain joint congruency while allowing for motion (Fig. 6.2). Static pinning or external fixation would be additional surgical options that would restore alignment, but these treatments would likely invite more stiffness than a dynamic construct. Because this patient had an intact dorsal cortex at the middle phalanx, a force couple device was an option. Without this intact cortex, another technique would need to be chosen.

Clinical Course and Outcome

The patient underwent placement of a force couple device (see pearls and pitfalls). Figure 6.3 outlines the procedure in stepwise and schematic form. Briefly, a 0.045 or 0.054 in. K-wire was passed parallel to the PIP joint through the head of the proximal phalanx at

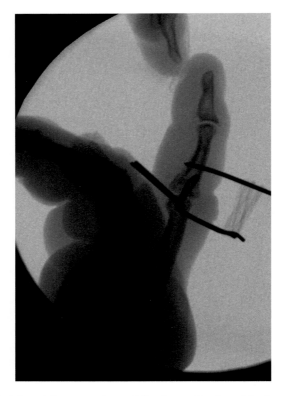

Fig. 6.2 A lateral fluoroscan image following application of the force couple device

➤

Fig. 6.3 (continued) middle phalanx is bent to allow passage volar to the proximal phalangeal K-wire. (**f**) The proximal phalangeal pin is bent volarly to secure and stabilize the middle phalangeal pin. (**g**) A small bend (shepherd's crook) at the ends of the middle phalanx pin will help stabilize the rubber band (**h**) which passes from the ends of the bend around the sagittal 0.062 threaded pin

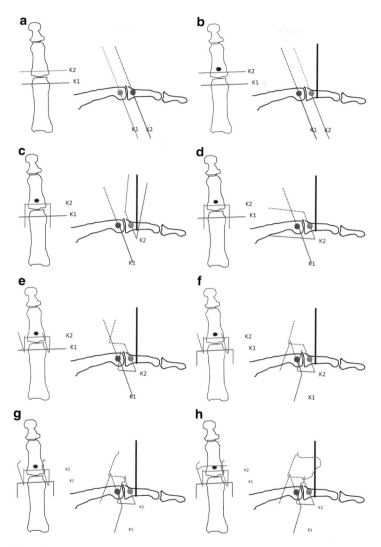

Fig. 6.3 (**a**) Two coronal place 0.045 K-wires are placed across the finger perpendicular to the long axis of the bones: one in the center of rotation of the proximal phalangeal head and another in the proximal aspect of the middle phalanx. (**b**) A sagittal plane threaded 0.062 K-wire is placed in a dorsal to volar direction of the middle phalanx. (**c–e**) The coronal plane K-wire in the

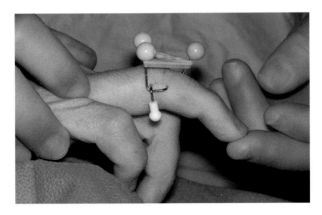

Fig. 6.4 An illustrative example of the completed construct of the force couple device on a patient

the center of rotation (K1). A second 0.045 or 0.054 in. K-wire (K2) was passed parallel to the PIP joint through the proximal aspect of the middle phalanx; this pin was passed just dorsal to the midline of the digit (K2). A dorsally to volarly directed 0.062 in. threaded K-wire was placed in the middle phalanx in the proximal half of the middle phalanx, distal to the transverse K-wire (K2). The limbs K2 were bent at 90°, leaving about the width of a needle driver on either side to allow swelling of the digit; the limbs of K2 were bent proximally and volarly to K1. A second bend was placed in the K2 limbs, this time 5–10 mm proximal to K1; the limbs were bent upward 90° and then each limb was fashioned into a "hook" dorsal to the finger. The limbs of K1 were bent 90° downward. A rubber band was placed over the hooks in K2 and about the threaded vertically directed K-wire, creating the force couple device. Figure 6.4 demonstrates the final construct and appearance.

After a brief period of immobilization, the patient was started on range-of-motion exercises at 4 days following surgery. He was advised to avoid getting the finger wet or dirty and instructed in pin care for the device. Progressive range of motion followed with the device in place. The force couple was removed at 7 weeks following surgery. Final radiographs revealed a healed fracture with congruent joint (Fig. 6.5a, b). At 6 months following surgery, flexion-extension arc of motion of the finger was 0–95 for the metacarpophalangeal

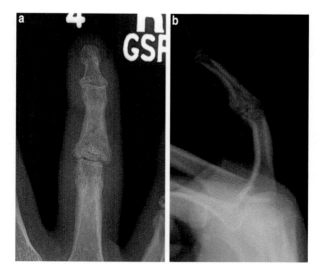

Fig. 6.5 (**a**) PA and (**b**) lateral X-rays following removal of the device demonstrate healed fracture and congruent joint

joint, 10–90 for the PIP joint, and 0–30 for the DIP joint. The pin sites healed uneventfully and he denied any numbness and tingling. Final grip strength of the hand was 40 kg (83 % of the contralateral side).

Clinical Pearls/Pitfalls

Pearls

- 0.045 or 0.054 in. K-wires generally are the best choice for proximal phalangeal and proximal middle phalangeal pins.
- A threaded 0.062 or 0.054 in. K-wire is the preferred choice for the dorsal middle phalangeal pin.
- It is important to place the proximal phalanx pin at the center of rotation of the condyles.
- Placing the proximal middle phalangeal joint pin slightly dorsal of the midline will help ensure that the joint reduces adequately and that the reduction is maintained.

- Fluoroscopy is essential in confirming appropriate reduction and pin placements and length.
- Bending the coronal plane pins such that they are close to the skin (by approximately the width of a large needle driver) will minimize irritation of the adjacent digits.
- A minimum of 6 weeks is appropriate to leave the fixator in place. The surgeon can release the rubber band and assess the finger fluoroscopically prior to removal of the pins to ensure the joint maintains its congruency through its arc of motion.
- Encourage early distal interphalangeal (DIP) joint motion early in the recovery to maximize motion at that joint.

Pitfalls

- This technique requires an intact dorsal cortex of the middle phalanx.
- Over-tensioning of the device with the rubber bands will limit finger flexion during the rehabilitation process.
- Another potential side effect to over aggressive rubber bands is the development of hyperextension of the PIP joint. Fluoroscopy can confirm this and early correction of the tension will correct this problem.
- It is important to follow these patients closely for pin monitoring to ensure that they are free of infection. Pins that are not precisely placed will also invite motion within the bone as well as at the skin and may be more vulnerable to pin tract infections.
- In addition, failure to closely monitor the patients radiographically can invite problems if the patient loses their reduction and continues to try and rehabilitate.

Literature Review and Discussion

PIP fracture-dislocations can result in significant morbidity to patients. Early identification and treatment provides the best hope for optimal outcomes. Because the bony constraints of the PIP joint are important stabilizers, the ideal treatment of fracture-dislocations is largely dependent on the extent of bony injury and locations of the fractures. Dorsal fracture-dislocations are the most common fracture pattern. Tyser et al. performed a cadaver study examining the stability of the PIP joint following incrementally larger fragment fractures of the volar aspect of the proximal middle phalangeal joint surface [1]. The authors noted that fractures involving 20 % or less of the articular surface were uniformly stable. In specimens with 40 % of the articular surface involvement, 28 % of these joint were unstable. All of the specimens with 60 and 80 % involvement were unstable.

These findings are consistent with our clinical experiences. McElfresh et al. examined outcomes of extension block splinting for dorsal PIP fracture-dislocations [2]. The authors noted that fractures from 10 to 30 % articular surface involvement were generally stable, while those from 30 to 50 % were more candidates for this method of treatment, and those greater than 50 % were less likely to be successfully treated with extension block splinting. Generally speaking most described techniques for splinting are initiated at the point of extension that affords congruency of the joint, which is usually 25–45°, and the splint is dialed back by approximately 10° per week.

Extension block pinning is a closed treatment that mimics the method of extension block splinting. A K-wire is used to block the PIP joint from extension and maintain joint congruency through the healing process. It has the advantage of being more dependable than splinting in maintaining the reduction. However, the downside is that you cannot dial it out over time. Maalla et al. examined their outcomes on 22 cases treated in this manner [3]. At an average 2.5-year follow-up period, the authors noted a mean arc of motion of 85° and good results in 82 % of patients.

Stern et al. published a study which nicely illustrates the complexity of managing these injuries [4]. The authors compared three treatments, splinting, open reduction, and skeletal traction, for pilon fractures of the PIP joint in 20 cases with 2-year follow-up interval. The authors felt that static splinting was undesirable and open reduction should be approached with caution and may result in significant complications. Skeletal traction was safer and provided radiographic results similar to open reduction.

The first skeletal traction and external fixation devices were static and were initially described by Robertson et al. [5]. These first descriptions were static, and over time, we have evolved to develop dynamic external fixators that allow for the advantage of motion while maintaining joint congruency. Agee was one of the first to publish a rationale and experience with what he described as a force couple device [6]. It had advantages over the previously published banjo frame described by Schenk which was large, bulky, and technically very demanding to place and maintain [7]. However, for the force couple to be predictably effective, it requires an intact dorsal column of the middle phalanx. Because the mechanism of maintaining the reduction is based more on a volar-directed vector on the joint and not by distraction per se, persons with a disrupted dorsal cortex of the middle phalanx (as seen in pilon fractures) are vulnerable to loss of reduction, hyperextension, or dorsal collapse of the joint when using the force couple device.

For pilon fractures and fracture-dislocations that involve the dorsal and volar columns of the middle phalanx, a number of other dynamic external fixation methods have been described with generally equally effective results [8–14]. These techniques are based on a longitudinal distraction force to maintain the joint congruency and therefore not as dependant on an intact dorsal cortex of the middle phalanx. Their indications also include cases where the dorsal column of the joint is intact. One of the more commonly utilized is the method described by Suzuki et al. [13]. It involves three K-wires placed in the coronal plane of the finger: one at the center of the condyles of the proximal phalanx, another at the proximal aspect of the middle phalanx (distal to the fracture), and the last in the distal aspect of the middle phalanx. Rubber band traction is set up between the proximal and distal wires, with the middle pin stabilizing the construct. The authors described excellent results on seven cases treated with this method, with congruent PIP joints and an 80° arc of PIP motion. In addition, the authors noted a DIP arc of motion of 0–40°. Similar results were experiences with the experience of Rutland et al. Thirty-four patients were treated, most were dorsal fracture-dislocations, six were pilon, and three were chronic (6 week average). Overall outcomes were excellent with a final arc of motion of 88° at 16-month follow-up. The average DIP arc was 60°. Eight cases of pin tract infections were noted, with all of them resolved with antibiotics. They concluded that this technique was good for both acute and chronic PIP fracture-dislocations.

Compass hinges have also been utilized for PIP fracture-dislocations. Krakauer and Stern reported their results using one of these devices on 20 cases. They subdivided the patients into those treated within 4 weeks (group 1) and those more than 4 weeks (group 2). The authors noted that while both groups fared well with regard to motion and overall pain, the acutely treated group had better outcomes [11].

Conclusion

Dorsal PIP fracture-dislocations can be difficult injuries to manage. The stability of the joint is dependent on the amount of volar articular disruption of the middle phalanx. Maintenance of joint congruency is essential to optimize outcomes. The fractures are often too comminuted for open reduction and internal fixation. When closed treatments are unsuccessful in maintaining joint congruency, the surgeon can consider the use of dynamic external fixation. The force couple device is a clever way to maintain joint congruency while allowing range of motion. When placed appropriately, excellent outcomes can be anticipated. Optimal results are achieved in patients with an intact dorsal column of the joint. The surgeon should consider other options in patients who do not have an intact dorsal cortex, in the chronic setting, and in patients who are unlikely to tolerate external devices.

References

1. Tyser AR, Tsai MA, Parks BG, et al. Stability of acute dorsal fracture dislocations of the proximal interphalangeal joint: a biomechanical study. J Hand Surg Am. 2014;39(1):13–8.
2. McElfresh EC, Dobyns JH, O'Brien ET. Management of fracture-dislocation of the proximal interphalangeal joints by extension-block splinting. J Bone Joint Surg Am. 1972;54(8):1705–11.

3. Maalla R, Youssef M, Ben Jdidia G, et al. Extension-block pinning for fracture-dislocation of the proximal interphalangeal joint. Orthop Traumatol Surg Res. 2012;98(5):559–63.

4. Stern PJ, Roman RJ, Kiefhaber TR, et al. Pilon fractures of the proximal interphalangeal joint. J Hand Surg Am. 1991;16(5):844–50.

5. Robertson RC, Cawley Jr JJ, Faris AM. Treatment of fracture-dislocation of the interphalangeal joints of the hand. J Bone Joint Surg Am. 1946;28: 68–70.

6. Agee JM. Unstable fracture dislocations of the proximal interphalangeal joint treatment with the force couple splint. Clinical Orthopaedics and Related Research 1987; (214):101–12.

7. Schenck RR. Dynamic traction and early passive movement for fractures of the proximal interphalangeal joint. J Hand Surg Am. 1986;11(6): 850–8.

8. Badia A, Riano F, Ravikoff J, et al. Dynamic interdigital external fixation for proximal interphalangeal joint fracture dislocations. J Hand Surg Am. 2005;30(1):154–60.

9. Hynes MC, Giddins GEB. Dynamic external fixation for pilon fractures of the interphalangeal joints. J Hand Surg Br. 2001;26B(2):122–4.

10. Inanami H, Ninomiya S, Okutsu I, et al. Dynamic external finger fixator for fracture dislocation of the proximal interphalangeal joint. J Hand Surg Am. 1993;18(1):160–4.

11. Krakauer JD, Stern PJ. Hinged device for fractures involving the proximal interphalangeal joint. Clin Orthop Relat Res. 1996;327:29–37.

12. Ruland RT, Hogan CJ, Cannon DL, et al. Use of dynamic distraction external fixation for unstable fracture-dislocations of the proximal interphalangeal joint. J Hand Surg Am. 2008;33(1):19–25.

13. Suzuki Y, Matsunaga T, Sato S, et al. The pins and rubbers traction system for treatment of comminuted intraarticular fractures and fracture-dislocations in the hand. J Hand Surg Br. 1994;19(1):98–107.

14. Ellis SJ, Cheng R, Prokopis P, et al. Treatment of proximal interphalangeal dorsal fracture-dislocation injuries with dynamic external fixation: a pins and rubber band system. J Hand Surg Am. 2007;32(8):1242–50.

Chapter 7
ORIF with Screw Fixation

Chris Lincoski

Abstract Open reduction and internal fixation is an option for treatment of PIP fracture-dislocations. The technique typically involves an open volar approach with placement of one or two 1.1–1.5 mm screws. This allows for restoration of the volar lip of the middle phalanx, which is the bony buttress to dorsal subluxation. The goal of fixation is to achieve a congruent joint and sufficient stability to allow for immediate active range of motion.

Keywords Proximal interphalangeal joint • Fracture-dislocation of proximal interphalangeal joint • Open reduction internal fixation • Mini-screw • Dislocation

Introduction

There are many options to treat PIP fracture-dislocations, including closed reduction and extension block splinting, extension block pinning, dynamic external fixation, and open reduction with

C. Lincoski, M.D. (✉)
Department of Orthopedic Hand Surgery, University Orthopedic Center,
101 Regent Court, State College, PA 16801, USA
e-mail: clincosk@gmail.com

© Springer International Publishing Switzerland 2016
J.E. Adams (ed.), *PIP Joint Fracture Dislocations*,
DOI 10.1007/978-3-319-28579-5_7

internal fixation. Open reduction and internal fixation is a means to achieve stability of the PIP joint when there is a large volar fracture fragment without substantial comminution.

Pathology

The volar lip of the middle phalanx provides a buttress to dorsal subluxation of the PIP joint. Loss of this bony buttress can result in instability of the PIP joint. Fractures involving less than 20 % of the joint surface are typically stable. Fractures involving greater than 40 % are unstable [1]. With fractures involving greater than 40 % of the articular surface, the majority of the volar plate and collateral ligaments remain attached to the fractured fragment, contributing to instability. If the fractured fragment is large, internal fixation can restore the bony buttress of the middle phalanx, restoring joint congruity and preventing joint subluxation.

Indications

The primary indication for ORIF of intra-articular PIP fractures is a large fracture fragment without substantial comminution that is associated with joint instability. The smaller the fractured piece, the harder it is to place screws. Comminution may preclude successful internal fixation. Typical indications include volar lip fractures with greater than 2 mm of displacement and joint instability with a fracture piece large enough to accommodate a screw [2].

Comminution of the fracture fragment is the main contraindication to internal fixation. The fragment should be at least twice the diameter of the intended screw hole. Typically 1.1–1.5 mm screws are used. Two screws are ideal to provide rotational control and increase stability [2, 3].

A large avulsion of the central slip is another indication for ORIF. This can be approached dorsally and the same principles of fixation can be applied. Ideally, two 1.5 or 1.1 mm screws can be used for fixation. Care should be taken not to inadvertently comminute the piece and to allow for sufficient bone distally in the fracture fragment so that the screws do not pull out.

Treatment

The primary goal of treatment of PIP fracture-dislocations is to restore a stable congruent joint. Secondary goals are to obtain articular congruity and anatomic alignment of the joint surface. It should be emphasized that the most important principle is to obtain a stable, concentric joint. Having an alternative plan such as K-wire external fixation or volar plate arthroplasty is wise, as the fracture not uncommonly proves to be more comminuted than expected.

If the volar fragment is large, restoration of the volar lip of the middle phalanx provides a buttress to subluxation of the PIP joint. This can be accomplished with open reduction and internal fixation using a 1.1–1.5 mm screw if the fragment shows minimal comminution. Ideally, ORIF should be stable enough to allow for immediate protected range of motion.

ORIF is typically performed through a volar incision, although a dorsal incision has been described [4]. A volar Bruner incision typically allows for adequate exposure. The Bruner incision can be based radially in the index and long fingers and ulnarly in the ring and small fingers in order to reduce hypersensitivity of the scar. Subsequently, the A3 pulley should be opened and the flexor tendons retracted in a radial direction. The distal C1 and proximal C3 pulley can also be incised to allow for exposure.

The collateral ligaments can be detached if necessary to help facilitate exposure. The volar plate should be left attached to the fracture fragment if possible, as it will help contribute stability to the PIP joint. If the volar plate is left attached, fracture alignment can be evaluated with fluoroscopy and evaluation of the cortical alignment of the volar middle phalanx, as the surgeon attempts to "key in" the fracture fragment. Alternatively, the volar plate can be longitudinally incised so the surgeon can visually inspect the joint reduction as described by Green [5].

If there is impaction of the subchondral bone, these fragments can be elevated with a freer elevator. Occasionally bone graft can be placed if there is a void after impacted fragments are elevated.

Temporary trans-articular pinning can be used as augmentation fixation if the joint is unstable after fixation; however this should be discouraged. The goal of fixation is to provide sufficient stability to allow for immediate active range of motion. However, Grant, et al. reported good results with temporary pinning of the PIP joint after ORIF [6].

With increasing comminution, Cerclage wire is an option for ORIF. Weiss reported on this technique with similar results [7].

Results

Limited studies are available with only retrospective reviews and case studies. No randomized trials have been performed in comparison with ORIF versus other techniques.

In a retrospective review of nine patients treated with ORIF of unstable dorsal fracture-dislocations of the PIP joint, Hamilton reported a 70° average arc of motion. They reported eight of nine patients with a flexion contracture [8]. There recommendation was to approach the procedure with caution, especially in fractures with comminution. The percentage of articular surface involvement averaged 56 % with a range from 20 to 75. Six joints had three or more fracture fragments. Postoperative rehabilitation was begun at 2–9 days after surgery and active range of motion was started. The patient was placed in a figure of eight splint to limit 5° of extension. Five patients were very satisfied, three were satisfied, and one was dissatisfied. The dissatisfied patient had recurrent subluxation of the PIP joint. Degenerative changes were noted in three of nine patients in follow-up, highlighting the challenging nature of these injuries.

Green et al. reported on two cases treated with ORIF of a large volar fragment. He demonstrated excellent results in both cases [5]. He recommended stabilization of the joint by ORIF to allow for immediate range of motion.

Grant reported on 3-year follow-up of a cohort of 14 patients treated with ORIF. Patients were treated both acutely and chronically with a 1.2 mm screw and temporary extension block pinning of the PIP joint. Average total PIP range of motion in the acute group was 100° and 86° in the chronic group. Longer delay from injury was associated with a lower ROM. Three patients had loss of reduction, all of which were in the chronic group. They noted good results in 79 % [6].

Lee and Teoh described a dorsal approach for ORIF of PIP fracture-dislocation. They had no recurrent subluxation. Mean PIP ROM was 85°. They concluded that a dorsal approach is technically easier and provides adequate exposure to the joint; however, in 4 of 12 fingers then had difficulty with reduction and required an additional volar incision [4].

Ikeda reported on 18 patients treated by ORIF with a low-profile mini-plate. Active PIP range of motion was 85°. Two patients developed flexor tendon adhesions and limited DIP motion [9].

Author's Preferred Technique/Case Example

Case

Athirty-three-year-old male sustained an injury to his left index finger when a tractor-trailer engine exploded as he was working on it. He noted immediate pain and deformity. He was seen in the emergency department where an attempt at reduction of the finger was performed.

Radiographs revealed an intra-articular fracture at the base of the middle phalanx. One large fragment was noted, involving approximately 45 % of the joint. The joint showed dorsal subluxation, with a positive V sign (Fig. 7.1). Given the dorsal subluxation of the PIP joint, surgical treatment was recommended. Nonoperative treatment was not recommended as it would likely lead to posttraumatic arthrosis and a stiff PIP joint, given the joint incongruity. Options for surgical treatment were discussed, including ORIF and K-wire external fixation. The fracture was one large piece without comminution, making it an ideal candidate for ORIF.

The patient was brought to the operating room, and a digital block and sedation was performed. Mini C-arm fluoroscopy confirmed

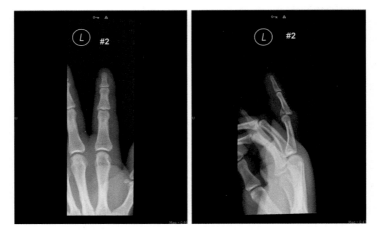

Fig. 7.1 (**a**) Preoperative PA and (**b**) lateral view demonstrate a PIP fracture-dislocation. Note the subluxation of the PIP joint and a single large fracture fragment

joint instability with dorsal dislocation of the PIP joint. The joint was reducible, but unstable. A volar Bruner approach was used and the neurovascular bundles were identified and protected. The A3 and C3 pulleys were incised and the flexor tendons were retracted in both a radial and ulnar direction to facilitate exposure. The volar plate was identified and was left attached to the fracture fragment. The fracture site was cleaned of debris. The fracture was manually reduced and held in place with a small pointed fracture reduction clamp while two holes were drilled to accept the two fixation screws. Two 1.2 mm screws were placed, one on each side of the fracture reduction clamp in a countersunk fashion (the author prefers to countersink the screws to prevent screw prominence and decrease the likelihood of screw cutout).

The joint was placed through a range of motion and stability of the joint was confirmed. The A3 pulley was repaired with 5-0 Monocryl. The volar plate was left attached to the fracture fragment and contributed to stability of the PIP joint.

The patient was splinted and started in hand therapy on post-op day 2. At that point, a hand-based splint with the PIP in slight flexion

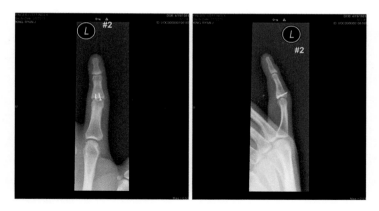

Fig. 7.2 Final postoperative radiographs at 5 months after surgery. (**a**) PA and (**b**) lateral radiographs demonstrate a congruent PIP joint with correction of joint subluxation. Slight step off in joint alignment is seen

was fabricated, and short arc AROM of the PIP joint was begun on post-op day 2.

At final follow-up, range of motion of the PIP joint was from 22 to 75°, highlighting the problems with stiffness after ORIF. Radiographs showed a healed fracture without joint incongruity or malalignment (Fig. 7.2). The patient was able to return to work as a laborer, but continued to have complaints of stiffness.

Conclusions

ORIF of PIP fracture-dislocations is a technically demanding procedure, best indicated for a single large fracture piece without comminution. The goals of fixation should be to achieve sufficient stability to allow for immediate active range of motion.

Technical Pearls If a 1.5 mm screw is used, a 1.1 mm K-wire (0.045 in.) is the same size as the drill bit used to place a 1.5 mm screw in a nonlag fashion. Two 1.1 mm K-wires can be placed in the fragment to stabilize it. One K-wire can be removed and a screw placed into that K-wire hole, while the second K-wire holds the bone stabilized. The second K-wire can then be likewise replaced with a screw. Likewise, if a 1.1 mm screw is used, a 0.7 mm (0.028 in.) K-wire can be used as a "drill."

Be very careful to avoid additional comminution of the bone. You get one good chance to place the screw. Take your time!

Countersinking the screws can help to minimize the chance of the screws breaking through the cortex.

If the volar plate is left intact, it is difficult to evaluate the joint reduction. If the piece is not comminuted, joint alignment can be approximated by aligning the distal cortical edges of the fracture.

References

1. Kiefhaber TR, Stern PJ. Fracture dislocations of the proximal interphalangeal joint. J Hand Surg Am. 1998;23A:368–80.
2. Freeland AE, Benoist LA. Open reduction and internal fixation method for fractures at the proximal interphalangeal joint. Hand Clin. 1994;10:239–50.
3. Jupiter JB, Sheppard JE. Tension wire fixation of avulsion fractures in the hand. Clin Orthop Relat Res. 1985;214:113–20.
4. Lee JY, Teoh LC. Dorsal fracture dislocations of the proximal interphalangeal joint treated by open reduction and interfragmentary screw fixation: indications, approaches and results. J Hand Surg Br. 2006;31:138–46.
5. Green A, Smith J, Redding M, Akelman E. Acute open reduction and rigid internal fixation of proximal interphalangeal joint fracture dislocation. J Hand Surg Am. 1992;17A:512–7.
6. Grant I, Berger AC, Tham SK. Internal fixation of unstable fracture dislocations of the proximal interphalangeal joint. J Hand Surg Br. 2005;30B:492–8.
7. Weiss AP. Cerclage fixation for fracture dislocation of the proximal interphalangeal joint. Clin Orthop Relat Res. 1996;327:21–8.
8. Hamilton SC, Stern PJ, Fassler PR, Kiefhaber TR. Mini-screw fixation for the treatment of proximal interphalangeal joint dorsal fracture-dislocations. J Hand Surg Am. 2006;31A:1349–54.
9. Ikeda M, Kobayashi Y, Saito I, Ishii T, Shimizu A, Oka Y. Open reduction and internal fixation for dorsal fracture dislocations of the proximal interphalangeal joint using a miniplate. Tech Hand Up Extrem Surg. 2011;15:219–24.

Chapter 8
Volar Plate Arthroplasty

O. Alton Barron and Daniel S. Donovan

Abstract Volar plate arthroplasty (VPA) is a treatment option for
comminuted and unstable dorsal fracture-dislocations of the proximal interphalangeal joint (PIP). The volar plate is reattached to the
volar edge of the remaining articular surface in order to provide a
restraint to dorsal subluxation and a smooth surface for articulation
with the head of the proximal phalanx.

In this chapter, VPA is discussed, including indications, anatomy
specific to the volar plate, technique, postoperative protocol, liter-
ature-based outcomes, and complications. A case is presented of
a dorsal fracture-dislocation of the proximal interphalangeal joint
treated by volar plate arthroplasty.

Keywords Fracture-dislocation • Proximal interphalangeal joint
• Volar plate arthroplasty • Palmar plate arthroplasty • Palmar plate
advancement • Volar plate advancement • Proximal interphalangeal
joint resurfacing arthroplasty

O.A. Barron, M.D. (✉)
Department of Orthopedics, CV Starr Hand Surgery Center, Mt. Sinai—
Roosevelt Hospital, Mt. Sinai Icahn School of Medicine, 1000 Tenth Avenue,
New York, NY 10019, USA
e-mail: oabarron@msn.com

D.S. Donovan, M.D.
Department of Orthopaedic Surgery, Mt. Sinai-St. Luke's Roosevelt,
New York, NY, USA

© Springer International Publishing Switzerland 2016   93
J.E. Adams (ed.), *PIP Joint Fracture Dislocations*,
DOI 10.1007/978-3-319-28579-5_8

Abbreviations

VPA   Volar plate arthroplasty
PIP   Proximal interphalangeal

Case

A healthy 29-year-old right-hand dominant male presented to the hand clinic with left fourth finger pain after catching a softball bare-handed and jamming his finger 1 week ago. He had presumed his injury was "a bad sprain" and had treated himself by buddy taping. On physical exam, his left fourth finger was swollen, bruised, and tender to palpation about the PIP with limited range of motion secondary to pain.

The lateral radiograph (Fig. 8.1) demonstrated a fracture of the base of the middle phalanx with 50 % volar articular damage and posterior subluxation.

The patient was counseled regarding the risks and benefits of surgery, and he agreed to proceed with surgery. The preoperative plan was to proceed with open reduction and internal fixation if the pieces were amenable to fixation or volar plate arthroplasty if the fragments were too comminuted for fixation.

Intraoperatively, the fracture was not able to be reduced and fixed secondary to comminution. Therefore, a decision was made to proceed with volar plate arthroplasty. Following the volar plate arthroplasty, a Kirschner wire driven across the PIP joint to fix the joint at 20° of flexion and a splint were applied.

At 2 weeks after surgery, the Kirschner wire was removed in the office, and the patient began range of motion exercises with extension block splinting. At 5 weeks, he continued to have a flexion contracture, and he began night extension splinting.

At 8 weeks, the patient had achieved a pain-free and stable 95° arc range of motion.

At 11-year follow-up, the joint remained reduced with stable range of motion, and the volar lip of the middle had partially reconstituted (Fig. 8.2).

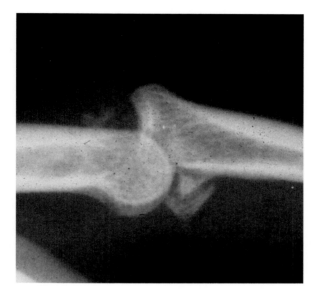

Fig. 8.1 Lateral radiograph of the PIP of the fourth digit demonstrates a fracture of the base of the middle phalanx with 50 % volar articular damage and posterior subluxation

Introduction

Volar fractures of the base of the middle phalanx disrupt both the bony buttress and soft tissue restraints to dorsal subluxation leading to instability. This also creates an irregular cartilage and subchondral surface articulating with the proximal phalanx. Introduced in 1967, the volar plate arthroplasty (VPA) has been a treatment option for comminuted and unstable dorsal fracture-dislocations of the proximal interphalangeal (PIP) joint. The volar plate is reattached to the volar edge of the remaining articular surface to provide a restraint to dorsal re-subluxation and a smooth surface for articulation with the head of the proximal phalanx. With the advent of various external and internal fixation techniques, the indications for VPA have narrowed; however, when performed for select indications

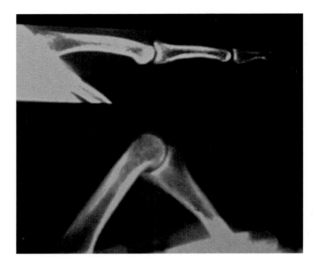

Fig. 8.2 Follow-up radiograph at 11 years demonstrates a nicely reconstituted volar lip of the middle phalanx (as can occur in a minority of cases)

with attention to technique, this procedure can provide pain relief, satisfactory restoration of motion, and joint stability.

Indications

Volar plate arthroplasty (VPA) is indicated for unstable dorsal fracture-dislocations of the proximal interphalangeal (PIP) joint, particularly in cases where comminution of the middle phalangeal volar base fracture is not amenable to anatomic open reduction and internal fixation. The reattachment of the volar plate to the middle phalanx provides stability as a static tether against dorsal subluxation and simultaneously resurfaces the joint [1].

Eaton originally described his indications for VPA as unstable acute fractures of the volar articular surface of the middle phalanx involving greater than 40 % of the surface; he later expanded his indications to include chronic instability [2]. VPA is useful to address volar lip fractures that are not amenable to open reduction and internal fixation. Prior to the introduction of autografting techniques such as hemihamate reconstruction [3], there were few if any good alternatives to VPA for greater amounts of PIP joint destruction [4]. Unpredictable clinical results of VPA by some authors helped to clarify and narrow the clinical indications for VPA [5–7]. Contraindications to VPA include abnormal contour or pathology of the proximal phalanx or a digit with poor vascularity [8].

Generally, better results including greater range of motion and decreased flexion contracture have been noted in younger patients, acute injuries, and injuries involving less of the joint surface [2]. However, many authors have published results of joint surface involvement from 30 to 40 % [7] to 50–90 % [6] (see Table 8.1). This author's preference is unstable fractures of 30–50 % of the volar articular middle phalanx with comminution precluding anatomic open reduction and internal fixation of the fragments. VPA performed with over 40 % articular involvement seems to have less predictable or worse results.

Table 8.1   Published indications for volar plate arthroplasty

30–40 % of articular surface	Ishida and Ikuta [7]
30–50 % of articular surface	Bednar et al. [9]
Greater than 40 % acute or chronic subluxation	Eaton and Malerich [2], Dionysian and Eaton [1]
Lower than or equal to 60 %	Malerich and Eaton [10]
Unstable dorsal fracture/dislocation, 50–70 %	Krakauer and Stern [11]
30–80 % of articular surface	Deitch et al. [5]
Salvage, 50–90 %	Hastings and Carroll [6]
Acute fracture/dislocation with comminution of volar lip, or chronic subluxation, no specific percent noted	Durham-Smith and McCarten [4], Bilos et al. [12], Lee et al. [13], Blazar et al. [8]

Anatomy of the Volar Plate

Successful volar plate arthroplasty relies on an understanding of the unique anatomic characteristics of the volar plate. The volar plate is composed of connective tissue including fibrocartilage; it originates proximally in a swallowtail configuration from the lateral margins of the proximal phalanx. This anatomic configuration prevents compression of blood supply to the vincular vessels which course under its attachments and contribute to the volar plate's role as a vascularized graft; these vessels must not be disrupted [14]. The vascular nature of this fibrocartilage pedicle not only supports its viability as a static graft but also has been hypothesized to promote bony remodeling of the volar middle phalanx [10].

Distally, the volar plate inserts on the volar metaphysis of the middle phalanx. The central tissue is less stout, taking a "meniscoid" configuration with the distal lateral insertion of the volar plate-collateral ligament complex acting as the primary static restraint to hyperextension in uninjured cadaveric specimens [14]. This highlights the importance of suture placement in the lateral edges of the volar plate, not in the center of the structure.

Technique

A volar Bruner (zigzag) incision is used with a radial-based flap, the apex at the level of the PIP joint. The dissection is carried down creating a full-thickness skin flap to the flexor sheath, which is incised between the A2 and A4 pulleys. The tendons are retracted [2].

Exploration and neurolysis of the digital nerves and arteries are not routinely required; however, some authors suggest exploring and freeing the bundle in chronic cases to prevent traction injury during joint exposure [10].

The fracture is evaluated with fluoroscopy and direct visualization. If the fragments are not amenable to anatomic fixation, they are excised from the volar plate and saved to be used as bone graft. The collateral ligaments are excised completely to facilitate exposure and

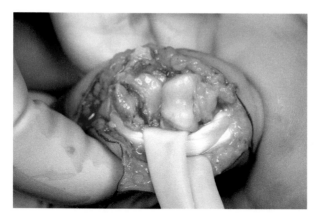

Fig. 8.3 The shotgun exposure to the joint demonstrates the articular damage

mitigate postoperative stiffness. The joint is then hyperextended in a "shotgun" fashion [10].

There is now a clear view of the articular damage (Fig. 8.3). Care must be taken to look for additional articular compression of the remaining articular surface. If present, this must be carefully disimpacted with a small osteotome and the wedge defect packed with allograft cancellous graft. Otherwise, the flattening of the articular contour will predispose to re-subluxation. A horizontal trough is created at the junction of the fracture and the remaining cartilage. The trough should be the dimensions of the end of the volar plate. The trough must be symmetric, or angular deformity will result (Fig. 8.4) [10].

A pullout wire or suture is passed through the lateral edges of the distal volar plate in a Kessler-type stitch or locking stitch of the surgeon's preference. Care must be taken to capture the thick tissue at the radial and ulnar aspect of the plate (Fig. 8.5). At this time, two drill holes are established, one at the radial aspect of the trough and one at the ulnar aspect of the trough. The holes should be drilled in a convergent fashion, yet exit the dorsal cortex before meeting each other in order to leave a bridge of cortical bone. The holes should be drilled and suture passed with the proximal and distal interphalangeal joints fully flexed to prevent entrapment of the extensor apparatus [15].

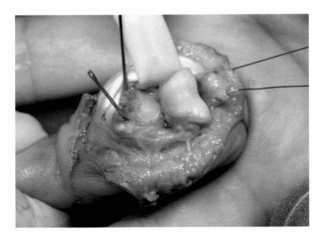

Fig. 8.4 An even, horizontal trough is established. In this image, the Keith needles have already been passed through the ulnar and radial aspects of the trough

If using a pullout wire (rare now), the wire is passed through their respective holes, and tension is drawn to reduce the volar plate to the fracture. Before tying the wire, the finger should be taken through a range of motion under fluoroscopy. If there is an unacceptable amount of flexion contracture, the proximal swallowtail ligaments may be sharply teased (fractionally lengthened) with the volar plate under tension to allow for increased distal excursion of the volar plate. If there is contracture limiting the ability of the finger to be brought into the palm, this may be addressed with dorsal capsular release, especially for chronic cases. Once satisfied with range of motion and stability, the pullout wire is tied over a button.

If using suture, after passage through the volar plate, it is passed through the drill holes with a Keith needle, and a small accessory incision is made dorsally between the lateral bands and the insertion of the central slip, so the knot may be tied deep to the extensor tendons (Fig. 8.6) [4].

If using suture anchors, suture is threaded through the anchor first and then passed through the volar plate, and stability and range of motion are judged [13]. Real-time pullout strength of the anchors must be judged since there is no cortical buttress to enhance pullout resistance.

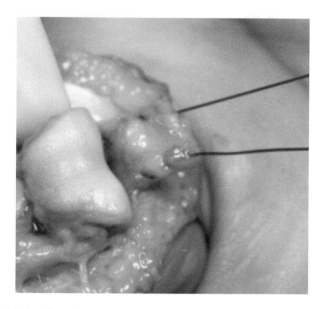

Fig. 8.5 A pullout wire or suture is passed through the lateral edges of the distal volar plate in a baseball, Kessler-type stitch or locking stitch capturing the thick tissue at the radial and ulnar aspect of the plate

After the suture or wire is tied, a Kirschner wire is driven across the dorsal aspect of the PIP joint with the joint in no greater than 30° of flexion to decrease risk of flexion contracture. Alternatively, a static or dynamic external fixator may be used. A true lateral on fluoroscopy must confirm reduction of the joint. A sterile dressing and splint are applied.

Evolution of Volar Plate Arthroplasty

In 1953, Moberg and Stener performed the first volar plate reattachment with a pullout wire [4], though this was not a resurfacing arthroplasty for fracture. In 1967, the first volar plate arthroplasty was performed by Richard Eaton, and he first reported this procedure in 1976 [16]. In 1980, he published his 10-year experience [2].

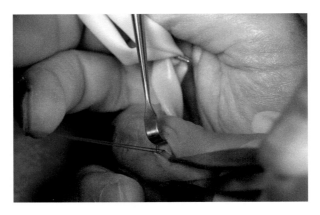

Fig. 8.6 Suture is passed through the drill holes and tied through a small accessory incision. The incision is placed dorsally between the lateral bands and the insertion of the central slip, so the knot may be tied deep to the extensor tendons

In 1992, Durham-Smith published a modification of the volar plate arthroplasty in which they did not release the collateral ligaments fully, nor did they use a full shotgun approach to the joint. Their modification included using a separate suture for each corner of the volar plate to avoid bunching of the plate, as well as tying the suture deep to the extensor apparatus to avoid skin complications [4]. In 1994, Bilos advocated for avoiding angulation of the digit by elevating depressed portions of the articular surface and fixation with Kirschner wires before performing the VPA. Additionally, Bilos modified the dorsal suture placement to tie directly on the triangular ligament through a dorsal incision [12]. In 1996, Krakauer published his use of a dynamic external fixator to encourage early return of motion [11]. In 1999, Deitch stressed the importance of backfilling the void in metaphyseal bone distal to the volar plate with bone graft or a slip of tendon. In 2000, Eaton and Dionysian published the long-term findings of the 33-year-old procedure [1]. In 2008, Lee published successful results of using suture anchors to perform VPA [13]. See Table 8.2 for the evolution of the VPA.

Table 8.2 The evolution of volar plate arthroplasty

1953	Volar plate reattachment not in presence of fracture—Moberg and Stener [4]
1967	First volar plate arthroplasty—Richard G Eaton [2]
1976	First published by Eaton and Littler [16]
1980	10-year experience published by Malerich and Eaton [2]
1992	Durham-Smith advocate against full release of collateral ligaments and full shotgun approach to joint. Use a separate suture for each corner to prevent bunching, and tie deep to the extensor tendons via small longitudinal incision on the dorsum of finger [4]
1994	Bilos recommends avoiding angulation by elevating depressed portions of the condyle and fixation with K-wires before performing VPA. Tie sutures dorsally directly on triangular ligament through dorsal approach [12]
1996	Krakauer publishes supplementing volar plate arthroplasty with dynamic external fixator [11]
2000	Long-term follow-up published [1]
2001	One suture with a Bunnell suture through both margins [8]
2008	Lee publishes the use of suture anchors [13]

Postoperative Care/Rehabilitation

The PIP joint is among the most susceptible to painful stiffness secondary to disuse and immobilization; however, the desire to mobilize this joint must be weighed against the concerns of disruption of the repair and dislocation or subluxation [17]. Many authors have proposed a variety of postoperative protocols, ranging from near-immediate range of motion in a dynamic external fixator [11] to Kirschner wire immobilization of up to 1 month post-op [5]. The most commonly used regimen, and our preference, is to remove the Kirschner wire immobilization at approximately 2 weeks to begin range of motion with extension block splinting. If pullout wire is used, it is removed at 3 weeks. If needed, dynamic extension splinting may begin at 5 weeks. See Table 8.3 for all published postoperative motion regimens.

Table 8.3 Postoperative regimen

	Authors
Time before K-wire removal (if applicable)	
2 weeks	Eaton and Malerich [2], Malerich and Eaton [10], Ishida and Ikuta [7], Dionysian and Eaton [1]
10 days	Durham-Smith and McCarten [4]
3 weeks	Bilos et al. [12], Blazar et al. [8]
28 days	Deitch et al. [5], Hastings and Carroll [6] (group 1)
Time to begin range of motion with extension block	
Immediate	Hastings and Carroll [6] (group 2)
2 weeks	Eaton and Malerich 80, Malerich and Eaton [10], Ishida and Ikuta 98, Dionysian and Eaton [1]
3 weeks	Glickel and Barron [15], Lee et al. [13]
10 days	Durham-Smith and McCarten [4]
Full active range of motion with dynamic extension splinting as needed	
4 weeks	Malerich and Eaton [10]
5 weeks	Eaton and Malerich [2], Ishida and Ikuta [7], Dionysian and Eaton [1], Krakauer and Stern [11] (remove hinge), Glickel and Barron [15]
6 weeks	Durham-Smith and McCarten [4], Lee et al. [13]

Literature-Based Outcomes

As with any technically challenging procedure and one that has been performed for disparate indications, there have been wide ranges of outcomes. In Eaton's original series, the acute cases (surgery less than 4 weeks after injury) averaged range of motion of 95° with a flexion contracture of 6°. The chronic cases (surgery 6 weeks to 2 years post injury) had an average range of motion of 78°, with a flexion contracture of 12°. The DIP joint had on average 10° loss of motion. Overall, the authors noted younger patients and acute cases tended to have superior outcomes [2].

Hastings reported on two groups, one in which the PIP joint was immobilized with a Kirschner wire postoperatively and one immobilized with an external fixator. Their indications for surgery were either as a salvage procedure or acutely in the setting of the destruction of the majority of the articular surface of the base of the middle phalanx. The percentage of joint involved ranged from 50 to 90 % with an average of 65 %. Their range of motion in the Kirschner wire group was 49° with a flexion contracture of 34°, with only two of six patients with acceptable results. The external fixator group had a range of motion of 65° with a flexion contracture of 24°. In this group, they had one patient with "good" results, four "fair," and two "failures" [6].

Durham-Smith reported the largest published series, consisting of 71 volar plate arthroplasties. The authors noted that eventual patient satisfaction reached 94 %. The authors did not include the exact ranges of motion of their patients but reported that 62/71 had an average range of motion of 60° at 4 weeks and 95° pain-free stable range of motion at 8 weeks. Four patients had a flexion contracture from 10° to 35° [4].

Bilos' series of 23 patients reported in 1994 had an average range of motion of 69° degrees with a flexion contracture of 22°. Patients reported varied subjective impairment. One reported they could not use the finger, one had moderate impairment, five had slight impairment, and four had no impairment. Five patients had no pain; six patients had mild pain on use [12].

Krakauer also reported subjective and objective results with his sample of five patients in addition to noting that his acute patients had a range of motion of 58° with an extensor contracture of 12°, and his chronic patients had a range of motion of 80° with no extensor contracture. Three patients had no pain, one had mild pain with heavy activity, and one had moderate to severe pain [11].

In Ishida's series of six VPA, it was noted that arthritic changes were present on four patients' follow-up radiographs. Grip strength was 90 % on the operative hand compared with the contralateral side. There were no patients with excellent results, one with good, four with fair, and one patient with poor results. The range of motion averaged 54° with a flexion contracture of 21° [7].

Deitch reported on the long-term (average of 46 months) results of 24 patients with dorsal fracture-dislocations with either VPA or ORIF. They observed that 96 % of patients had little to no pain, 75 % had no difficulty with work, and there was no statistical difference between the range of motion in the VPA and ORIF groups [5].

Dionysian reported on the long-term results of 17 patients at an average of 11.5 years. No patients complained of pain at rest or with activity. Arthroplasty acutely after injury (less than 4 weeks) averaged active range of motion of 85° and extension lag of 15° with DIP range of motion of 58°. Chronic intervention (average 20 weeks) averaged 61° of active range of motion and 29° of extension lag and 28° of DIP motion. All patients returned to their original occupation and recreational activities. The two oldest patients, aged 59 and 61, had poor motion with only 30° and 50°. All patients had stable PIP joints to manual stress. Interestingly, in 90 % of the acute surgical patients, the volar lip of the middle phalanx underwent remodeling to reconstitute varying degrees of the volar lip, without backfill grafting at the time of surgery [1].

Lee reported a series of 20 patients treated with VPA with suture anchors. After an average follow-up of 25 months, the average range of motion was 82°. When broken into acute and chronic, the average range of motion was 93.6° for the acute group and 70.8° for the chronic group. The acute group had an average extension lag of 11.8°, whereas the chronic group had 20.9°. There was no reported rest or activity-related pain. At follow-up, 20 % of patients had joint remodeling that was similar to the adjacent non-injured finger [13].

See Table 8.4 for published postoperative range of motion.

Table 8.4   Average postoperative range of motion

Author	Postoperative average range of motion	Flexion contracture
Eaton and Malerich [2]	Acute: 95°	Acute: 6°
	Chronic: 78°	Chronic: 12°
Hastings and Carroll [6]	K-wire group: 49°	K-wire group: 34°.
	External fixator group: 65°	External fixator group: 24°
Durham-Smith and McCarten [4]	62/71 had average 60° at 4 weeks and 95° pain-free stable ROM at 8 weeks	Four patients had flexion contracture from 10° to 35°; the remainder were less
Bilos et al. [12]	69°	Flexion contracture 22°
Krakauer and Stern [11]	Acute: 58°	Acute:12°
	Chronic 80°	Chronic: no flexion contracture
Ishida and Ikuta [7]	54°	21°
Deitch et al. [5]	72°	8°
Dionysian and Eaton [1]	Acute: 85°	Acute: 15°.
	Chronic: 61°	Chronic: 29°.
Lee et al. [13]	Acute: 93.6°	Acute: 11.8°.
	Chronic 70.8°	Chronic: 20.9°

Complications

Complications reported after volar plate arthroplasty include redisplacement, flexion contracture, extensor adherence, angulation, infection, and dorsal skin necrosis. Steps may be taken to decrease the incidence of many of these complications.

Redisplacement has been reported at rates of 4 % [2], 31 % [6], and 20 % [11]; however, there have been have a number of series in which no redisplacement is noted [1, 4, 5, 7, 12, 13]. The risk of redisplacement may be decreased by ensuring proper reduction on fluoroscopy intraoperatively. Multiple authors also recommend filling the gap volar and distal to the volar plate with bone graft or a slip of FDS [5, 10], although it is not clear that this affects outcomes or even bone reconstruction.

Some degree of flexion contracture is inherent in VPA; a static structure is attached to a nonanatomic, more distal position. Furthermore, a certain degree of flexion is preferred to hyperextension, which would destabilize the joint. Series have reported flexion contracture from 0 to 34 %. Taking the joint through a range of motion before tying the sutures to secure the volar plate may minimize this risk. If there is an unacceptable amount of contracture, the proximal check-reign ligaments may be sharply teased to fractionally lengthen them and to functionally lengthen the volar plate.

Extensor adherence in one patient of Eaton's series required reoperation. One technical consideration to avoid this complication is to maximally flex the PIP and DIP while drilling through the middle phalanx and passing the sutures to avoid encountering the extensor mechanism [2].

Angulation has been observed in 12.5 % [2], 4 % [12], 18 % [1], and 35 % [13] as well as not reported [4–7, 11]. A technical aspect that prevents this pitfall is creating a symmetric trough in the middle phalanx into which to draw the volar plate. Restoring and backfilling any depressed remaining articular segments may also avoid this complication.

Infection has been seen in 15 % [6], 1.4 % [4], and 20 % [11] of cases as well as not reported by many authors [1, 2, 5, 7, 12, 13].

Dorsal skin necrosis was reported by one observer, at a rate of 4 % [4]. This may be avoided by making a dorsal accessory incision and tying suture below the skin rather than over a button, by taking additional care when tying over a button or using suture anchors.

See Table 8.5 for complications and prevention measures.

Summary

Since 1967, volar plate arthroplasty has remained a valuable treatment option with narrower indications for acute dorsal fracture-dislocations of the PIP joint as well as for cases of chronic instability and as a salvage procedure in the event of prior treatment

Table 8.5 Complications and prevention measures

Complication reported	Rate and series	Prevention measures [10]
Redislocation	4 % [2], 31 % [6], 20 % [11]	Ensure adequate immobilization post-op. May fill gap behind advanced volar plate with bone graft or a slip of FDS
Flexion contracture	See Table 8.4	Avoid splinting in excessive flexion, begin dynamic extension splinting before 6 weeks
Extensor adherence	4 % [2]	Flex DIP and PIP while passing pullout suture to avoid entrapment of lateral bands
Angulation	12.5 % [2], 4 % [12], 18 % [1], 35 % [13]	Create a symmetric trough
Infection	15 % [6], 1.4 % [4], 20 % [11]	Preoperative antibiotics, standard infection control measures
Dorsal skin necrosis	4 % [4]	Tie beneath the skin or use care when tying sutures over button

failure. The optimal candidate for volar plate arthroplasty is a patient with an unstable, comminuted, dorsal fracture-dislocation of 30–40 % (but up to 50 %) of the volar lip of the base of the middle phalanx. Though complications such as redisplacement and flexion contracture have been reported, these are more likely in chronic or salvage scenarios and can be avoided or mitigated by following the principles noted above. With such care to avoid complications and with attention to technique, satisfactory or better outcomes can be expected for these most complex and confounding injuries to the PIP joint.

References

1. Dionysian E, Eaton R. The long-term outcome of volar plate arthroplasty of the proximal interphalangeal joint. J Hand Surg Am. 2000;25(3): 429–37.

2. Eaton RG, Malerich MM. Volar plate arthroplasty of the proximal interphalangeal joint: a review of ten years' experience. J Hand Surg Am. 1980;5(3):260–8.

3. Calfee RP, Sommerkamp TG. Hemi-hamate arthroplasty provides functional reconstruction of acute and chronic proximal interphalangeal fracture-dislocations. J Hand Surg Am. 2009;34(7):1140–7.

4. Durham-Smith G, McCarten GM. Volar plate arthroplasty for closed proximal interphalangeal joint injuries. J Hand Surg Br. 1992;17B:422–8.

5. Deitch MA, Kiefhaber TR, Comisar R, Stern P. Dorsal fracture dislocations of the proximal interphalangeal joint: surgical complications and long-term results. J Hand Surg Am. 1999;24(5):914.

6. Hastings II H, Carroll IV C. Treatment of closed articular fractures of the metacarpophalangeal and proximal interphalangeal joints. Hand Clin. 1998;4(3):503–27.

7. Ishida O, Ikuta Y. Results of treatment of chronic dorsal fracture-dislocations of the proximal interphalangeal joints of the fingers. J Hand Surg Br. 1998;23(6):798–801.

8. Blazar PE, Robbe R, Lawton JN. Treatment of dorsal fracture/dislocations of the proximal interphalangeal joint by volar plate arthroplasty. Tech Hand Up Extrem Surg. 2001;5(3):148–52.

9. Bednar MS, Janelle C, Light T. Volar plate arthroplasty of the proximal interphalangeal joint. Oper Tech Orthop. 1996;6(2):117–20.

10. Malerich MM, Eaton RG. The volar plate reconstruction for fracture-dislocation of the proximal interphalangeal joint. Hand Clin. 1994;10(2):251–60.

11. Krakauer JD, Stern PJ. Hinged device for fractures involving the proximal interphalangeal joint. Clin Orthop Relat Res. 1996;327:29–37.

12. Bilos ZJ, Vender MI, Bonavolonta M, Knutson K. Fracture subluxation of proximal interphalangeal joint treated by palmar plate advancement. J Hand Surg Am. 1994;19(2):189–95.

13. Lee LS, Lee HM, Hou HT, Hung ST, Chen JK, Shih JT. Surgical outcome of volar plate arthroplasty of the proximal interphalangeal joint using the Mitek micro GII suture anchor. J Trauma. 2008;65(1):116–22.

14. Bowers WH, Wolf JW, Nehil JL, Bittinger S. The proximal interphalangeal joint volar plate. I. An anatomic and biochemical study. J Hand Surg Am. 1980;5(1):79–88.

15. Glickel SZ, Barron OA. Proximal interphalangeal joint fracture dislocations. Hand Clin. 2000;16(3):333–44.

16. Eaton RG, Littler JW. Joint injuries and their sequelae. Clin Plast Surg. 1976;3(1):85–98.

17. Littler JW, Thompson J. Dressings and splints. In: Converse's reconstructive plastic surgery, vol. 6. 2nd ed. Philadelphia, PA: Saunders; 1977.

Chapter 9
Pilon Fracture of the Proximal Interphalangeal Joint: Use of a Combination of Fixation Techniques

Elspeth Kinnucan

Abstract Proximal interphalangeal joint pilon fractures are unstable injuries with the potential sequelae of joint pain and stiffness. The goals for surgical treatment of these injuries are to create a stable, congruent joint with fixation that allows early motion as the fracture heals. This chapter presents the case of a proximal interphalangeal joint pilon fracture that was treated with dynamic external fixation, limited open reduction and internal fixation, and extension block pinning. By combining traction with direct reduction and fixation, satisfactory reduction of the joint was achieved, and the result was functional range of motion of the joint with minimal discomfort. This case suggests that surgeons become familiar with multiple treatment techniques for these injuries and be flexible in combining these techniques as required for individual fracture patterns.

Keywords Pilon • Fracture • Dislocation • Interphalangeal • Dynamic • External fixation • Pins and rubbers • Traction • Extension block pin • Internal fixation

E. Kinnucan, M.D. (✉)
Department of Orthopaedic Surgery, Kaiser Permanente,
1600 Eureka Rd, Roseville, CA 95661, USA
e-mail: Elspeth.X.Kinnucan@kp.org

Case

This 54-year-old, right-hand dominant man sustained an injury to the right small finger while using a drill. Initially, he thought that he had just "jammed" the finger and did not seek immediate medical attention. Two weeks after the injury, he presented for evaluation of persistent finger pain and swelling.

On examination, there was swelling about the proximal interphalangeal (PIP) joint of the right small finger. The skin was intact and there was no neurovascular injury. Radiographs revealed a pilon fracture of the right small finger proximal interphalangeal joint (Fig. 9.1). Surgical management of the injury was recommended.

The procedure was performed with an axillary block and monitored anesthesia care. A pneumatic arm tourniquet was used. First, a fluoroscopic view under traction was obtained, showing continued dislocation of the dorsal fracture fragment (Fig. 9.2). A dynamic

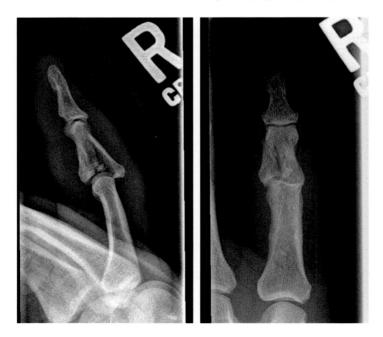

Fig. 9.1 Radiographs of the right small finger at the time of presentation

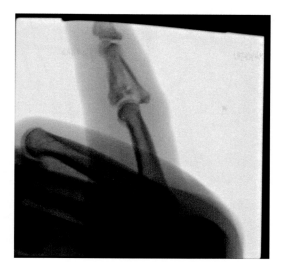

Fig. 9.2 Traction under fluoroscopy in the operating room

external fixator was applied utilizing 0.045-in. K-wires and rubber bands, as described by Slade et al. [1]. The middle phalanx diaphyseal wire could not be placed due to extension of the fracture, and the dorsal lip fragment remained dorsally dislocated. Therefore, a mini-open reduction was performed through the interval between the lateral band and central slip. The impacted joint fragments and dorsal lip fragment were reduced with a freer elevator. Two 0.035-in. K-wires were then placed across the base of the middle phalanx. Because of concern for potential joint subluxation, a 0.045-in. K-wire was placed in a retrograde fashion into the dorsal proximal phalanx as an extension block pin to further stabilize the dorsal fragment (Fig. 9.3). This fixation was a modification of the technique described by Vitale et al. [2] The result was a stable, congruent proximal interphalangeal joint throughout a range of motion.

Hand therapy was initiated at 5 days postoperatively. The patient had a hand-based thermoplastic splint fabricated and was instructed in pin care and active range of motion of the small finger proximal interphalangeal joint. The joint reduction was monitored radiographically with serial examination; clinical examination confirmed absence of pin tract infection or loosening of the pins and that the patient

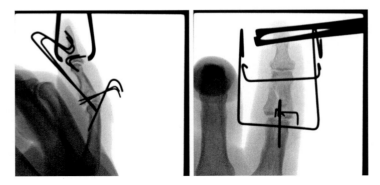

Fig. 9.3 Fluoroscopic views of the joint reduction and fixation, taken during surgery

continued to gain motion. At 6 weeks postoperatively, the external fixator and K-wires were removed. The patient was discharged from hand therapy at 10 weeks postoperatively. Radiographically, the fracture had healed, and the proximal interphalangeal joint remained congruent (Fig. 9.4). At final follow-up 15 months postoperatively, the patient reported occasional pain (1-2/10) with activity, good motion, and no functional limitations (Fig. 9.5). There were no tenderness or swelling in the finger. The proximal interphalangeal joint had 88° of flexion and lacked 18° of full extension. Distal interphalangeal joint flexion was 25°, with full active extension at this joint. There was 109 lb of grip strength in the right hand compared with 127 lb in the left hand. Final radiographs showed remodeling of the base of the middle phalanx and narrowing of the proximal interphalangeal joint (Fig. 9.6).

Introduction

Injuries to the proximal interphalangeal joint often prove to be challenging for both the patient and the providers treating them. The location of the proximal interphalangeal joint within the digit makes it susceptible to "jamming" injuries, where an axial force is applied to the extended digit [3]. Athletes participating in

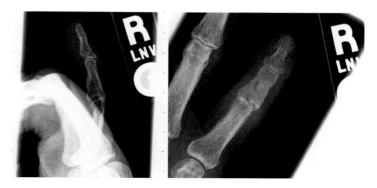

Fig. 9.4 Follow-up radiographs at 10 weeks postoperatively

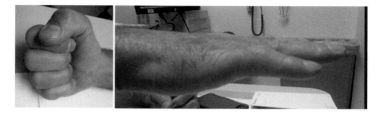

Fig. 9.5 Photographs of the right small finger flexion and extension at the final visit, 15 months after surgery

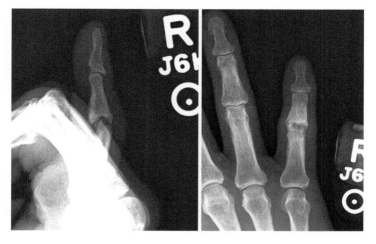

Fig. 9.6 Final radiographs at 15 months postoperatively

contact and ball-catching sports are particularly susceptible [4]. The proximal interphalangeal joint is responsible for 85 % of the finger motion needed for grasp [5]. Therefore, the possible long-term effects of these injuries, including pain, swelling, deformity, and loss of motion, can lead to significant dysfunction in the hand [6, 7, 8].

Pilon Fractures

Pilon fractures of the proximal interphalangeal joint occur with axial compression of the digit, causing joint impaction and fracture of both the volar and dorsal articular surfaces [10, 15]. The capsuloligamentous structures may remain intact. Pilon fractures are typically classified as either stable through full range of motion or as unstable [13].

The goals of treatment of pilon fractures are to achieve fracture union and maintain a stable, congruent joint that functions with a gliding rather than hinging motion [3, 9, 13]. Several authors note that allowing the joint to heal with a small articular step-off does not necessarily preclude a desirable outcome [11, 16]. The rehabilitation goals are to restore a functional range of motion and grip strength with minimal pain in the injured joint.

Treatment options for pilon fractures include splinting, open reduction and internal fixation, static external fixation, and dynamic external fixation [14, 15]. Nonsurgical management of pilon injuries is problematic unless the injury is axially stable [6]. Stern et al. found unsatisfactory results with splint management in four patients with pilon fractures of the proximal interphalangeal joint [15]. Dynamic external fixation is frequently the fixation technique of choice in pilon fractures. The traction reduces and stabilizes the comminuted joint surface and allows early motion of the joint. Open reduction and internal fixation of pilon fractures is indicated if the joint cannot be reduced with traction. Static external fixation of the proximal interphalangeal joint is indicated if there is significant bone loss or soft tissue injury that would preclude the other fixation options [12].

Dynamic External Fixation

The goal of dynamic external fixation is to maintain the proximal interphalangeal joint in satisfactory alignment and to allow early motion while the fracture heals. This technique relies on ligamentotaxis to reduce and stabilize the joint. The traction counteracts the deforming forces of the tendons and the shortening of the capsuloligamentous structures [1, 12]. The early motion reduces joint stiffness, improves tendon gliding, and promotes cartilage healing [17, 18].

Many different dynamic external fixation devices have been utilized for proximal interphalangeal joint injuries [1, 9, 12, 19]. The pin and rubber traction system is one of the most popular techniques due to the relative ease of application and readily available materials. The studies of dynamic external fixation of the proximal interphalangeal joint are limited to small retrospective reviews. However, many studies report functional ranges of motion when treating fracture-dislocation and pilon injuries of the proximal interphalangeal joint with dynamic external fixation [16, 20–31].

Table 9.1 summarizes published studies on the outcomes of dynamic external fixation for pilon fractures of the proximal interphalangeal joint. The average final motion of the proximal interphalangeal joint is fairly consistent thought the studies, 87–98° of flexion and 8–13° loss of extension reported. All of the studies had subjects with proximal interphalangeal joint pain at final follow-up. The rates of infection and radiographic evidence of arthritis were some what variable.

Open Reduction and Internal Fixation

The goal of open reduction and internal fixation of pilon fractures is to restore the articular surface and axial stability in the middle phalanx. Relatively little is written about this technique. Stern et al. reported on open reduction and internal fixation with K-wires in nine patients with pilon fractures of the proximal interphalangeal joint. The average period of immobilization was 4

Table 9.1 A summary of retrospective reviews of proximal interphalangeal joint pilon fractures treated with dynamic external fixation

Study	Number of subjects	Number of pilon fractures	Method of fixation	Mean follow-up (months)	Mean PIP motion (degrees)	Pain (number of subjects)	Arthritis (number of subjects)	Infection (number of subjects)
Hynes [20]	8	8	DEF	8	12–88	3	N/A	2
Syed [21]	8	9	DEF	26	8–87	1	1	0
Sarris [22]	6	6	DEF+ORIF	29	8–98	3	2	1
Mansha [23]	11	11	DEF	4	13–87	3	N/A	0

PIP proximal interphalangeal joint, *N/A* not available, *DEF* dynamic external fixation, *ORIF* open reduction and internal fixation

week. The average proximal interphalangeal joint flexion was 80°, and the average loss of extension was 10°. Seven of the nine patients reported pain at an average follow-up of 27 months. All of the patients lacked anatomic reduction of the joint surface. The authors concluded that it is difficult to achieve stable articular fixation adequate for early motion after open reduction and internal fixation of pilon fractures [15].

Other authors have combined dynamic external fixation and open reduction, with or without internal fixation of the fracture fragments [22, 24, 26, 28, 30]. The "mini-open" approach is often favored to limit the risks of scar tissue formation, infection, and devitalization of small fracture fragments.

Watanabe et al. looked at the factors that affect the functional results of open reduction and internal fixation of fractures and fracture-dislocations at the proximal interphalangeal joint. The study included 22 patients with pilon fractures and 38 patients with fracture-dislocations. K-wires were utilized for fixation in the majority of cases. They report an average proximal interphalangeal joint flexion of 78° and an average loss of extension of 11.5°. The factors affecting functional outcomes in these patients were a delay in active motion, elderly age, and ulnar digits [32]. This study further supports the need for early motion following treatment of these injuries, regardless of the fixation technique.

Extension Block Pinning

Traditionally, extension block pinning is employed when there is a comminuted fracture at the volar base of the middle phalanx and dorsal subluxation of the middle phalanx. The goal of the extension block pin is to prevent approximately 30° of proximal interphalangeal joint extension, thereby maintaining a congruent proximal interphalangeal joint and allowing motion of the joint.

Although this technique is not typically described for the treatment of pilon fractures of the proximal interphalangeal joint, use of this technique in combination with others may prove helpful [2, 33].

Complications

Stiffness is the most common complication resulting from injury to the proximal interphalangeal joint. Mild flexion contracture of the proximal interphalangeal joint is almost universal and should be combated with edema control, early motion, and splinting if necessary [34]. Several authors note that rehabilitation after surgery must focus on both the proximal and distal interphalangeal joints [1, 26, 34]. Loss of distal interphalangeal joint motion is commonly seen after both dynamic external fixation and open reduction and internal fixation, and stiffness of the distal interphalangeal joint contributes to disability in the digit.

Infection, pain, loss of reduction, joint instability, osteolysis, and pin loosening are also reported complications [34]. Nonunion is rarely an issue in these injuries.

Post-traumatic arthritis is always a concern when treating intra-articular fractures of the proximal interphalangeal joint. Subluxation and joint depression have been identified as risks for the development of post-traumatic arthritis [35]. However, several authors note that there is remodeling of the proximal interphalangeal joint, and when arthritis develops, it is not universally symptomatic [15, 16, 22, 25, 35, 36]. There does appear to be some tolerance for nonanatomic restoration of the base of the middle phalanx joint surface as long as the joint is congruent.

Conclusions for This Case

The challenge of this case was to create a stable, congruent joint that would withstand an early motion rehabilitation protocol. Dynamic external fixation is often the treatment of choice in pilon fracture of the proximal interphalangeal joint. Unfortunately, the dorsal lip fragment remained dislocated after traction was applied. Although open reduction was necessary, the use of a mini-open approach reduced the risks of scar tissue formation and devitalization of the fracture fragments. Rigid internal fixation may have been difficult to achieve given the comminution and impaction at the joint and would have required a more open approach. Because the dorsal lip fragment had a similar position to a dorsal fracture-dislocation, K-wire fixation and extension block pinning were chosen. The traction off-loaded the joint, and the interfragmentary K-wires and extension block pin stabilized the dorsal fragment. The early motion rehabilitation in this case reduced adhesions about the joint and improved tendon gliding in this digit. Final function and radiographic outcomes were satisfactory for this patient.

References

1. Slade JF, Baxamusa TH, Wolfe SW. External fixation of proximal interphalangeal joint fracture-dislocations. Atlas Hand Clin. 2000;5(1):1–29.
2. Vitale MA, White NJ, Strauch RJ. A percutaneous technique to treat unstable dorsal fracture-dislocation of the proximal interphalangeal joint. J Hand Surg Am. 2011;36(9):1453–9.
3. Shah CM, Sommerkamp TG. Fracture dislocation of the finger joints. J Hand Surg Am. 2014;39(4):709–802.
4. Williams C. Proximal interphalangeal joint fracture dislocations: stable and unstable. Hand Clin. 2012;28:409–16.
5. Leibovic SJ, Bowers WH. Anatomy of the proximal interphalangeal joint. Hand Clin. 1994;10(2):169–78.
6. Glickel SZ, Barron OA. Proximal interphalangeal joint fracture dislocations. Hand Clin. 2000;16:333–44.
7. Calfee RP, Sommerkamp MD. Fracture dislocation about the finger joints. J Hand Surg Am. 2009;34:1140–7.
8. Freiberg A. Management of proximal interphalangeal joint injuries. Can J Plast Surg. 2007;15(4):199–203.
9. Haase SC, Chung KC. Current concepts in treatment of fracture-dislocations of the proximal interphalangeal joint. Plast Reconstr Surg. 2014;134(6):1246–57.
10. Seno N, Hashizue H, Inoue H, Imatani J, Morito Y. Fractures of the base of the middle phalanx of the finger. Classification, management and long-term results. J Bone Joint Surg Br. 1997;79(5):758–63.
11. Kang R, Stern PJ. Fracture dislocations of the proximal interphalangeal joint. J Am Soc Surg Hand. 2002;2(2):47–59.
12. Liodaki E, Xing SG, Mailaender P, Stang F. Management of difficult intra-articular fracture or fracture dislocations of the proximal interphalangeal joint. J Hand Surg Eur Vol. 2015;40(1):16–23.
13. Elfar J, Mann T. Fracture-dislocations of the proximal interphalangeal joint. J Am Acad Orthop Surg. 2013;21:88–98.

14. Ng CY, Oliver CW. Fractures of the proximal interphalangeal joints of the fingers. J Bone Joint Surg Br. 2009;91:705–12.
15. Stern PJ, Roman RD, Kiefhaber TR, McDonough JJ. Pilon fractures of the proximal interphalangeal joint. J Hand Surg Am. 1991;16(5):844–50.
16. Morgan JP, Gordon DA, Klug MS, Perry PE, Barre PS. Dynamic digital traction for unstable comminuted intra-articular fracture-dislocations of the proximal interphalangeal joint. J Hand Surg Am. 1995;20(4):565–73.
17. Salter RB. The physiologic basis of continuous passive motion for articular cartilage healing and regeneration. Hand Clin. 1994;10(2):211–9.
18. Joyce KM, Joyce CW, Conroy F, Chan J, Buckley E, Carroll SM. Proximal interphalangeal joint dislocations and treatment: an evolutionary process. Arch Plast Surg. 2014;41(4):394–7.
19. Suzuki Y, Matsunaga T, Sato S, Yokoi T. The pins and rubbers traction system for treatment of comminuted intraarticular fractures and fracture-dislocations in the hand. J Hand Surg Br. 1994;19(1):98–107.
20. Hynes MC, Giddins GEB. Dynamic external fixation for pilon fractures of the interphalangeal joints. J Hand Surg Br. 2001;26(2):122–4.
21. Syed AA, Agarwal M, Boome R. Dynamic external fixator for pilon fractures of the proximal interphalangeal joints: a simple fixator for a complex fracture. J Hand Surg Br. 2003;28(2):137–41.
22. Sarris I, Goitz RJ, Sotereanos DG. Dynamic traction and minimal internal fixation for thumb and digital pilon fractures. J Hand Surg Am. 2004;29(1):39–43.
23. Mansha M, Miranda S. Early results of a simple distraction dynamic external fixator in management of comminuted intra-articular fractures of the base of the middle phalanx. J Hand Microsurg. 2013;5(2):63–7.
24. Ruland RT, Hogan CJ, Cannon DL, Slade JF. Use of dynamic distraction external fixation for unstable fracture-dislocations of the proximal interphalangeal joint injuries. J Hand Surg Am. 2008;33:19–25.
25. Ellis SJ, Cheng R, Prokopis P, Chetboun C, Wolfe SW, Athanasian EA, et al. Treatment of proximal interphalangeal dorsal fracture-dislocation injuries with dynamic external. J Hand Surg Am. 2007;32(8):1242.
26. Agarwal AK, Karri V, Pickford MA. Avoiding pitfalls of the pins and rubbers traction technique for fractures of the proximal interphalangeal joint. Ann Plast Surg. 2007;58:489–95.
27. Kiral A, Erken HY, Akmaz I, Yidirim C, Erler K. Pins and rubber band traction for treatment of comminuted intra-articular fractures of the hand. J Hand Surg Am. 2014;39(4):696–705.
28. Badia A, Riano F, Ravikoff K, Khouri R, Gonzalez-Hernandez E, Orbay JL. Dynamic intradigital external fixation for proximal interphalangeal joint fracture dislocations. J Hand Surg Am. 2005;30(1):154–60.
29. Allison DM. Fractures of the base of the middle phalanx treated by a dynamic external fixation device. J Hand Surg Br. 1996;21:305–10.
30. Finsen V. Suzuki's pins and rubber traction for fractures of the base of the middle phalanx. J Plast Surg Hand Surg. 2010;44:209–13.

31. Deshmukh SC, Kumar D, Mathur K, Thomas B. Complex fracture-dislocations on the proximal interphalangeal joint of the hand: results of a modified pins and rubbers traction system. J Bone Joint Surg Br. 2004;86:406–12.
32. Watanabe K, Kino Y, Yajima H. Factors affective the functional results of open reduction and internal fixation for fracture-dislocations of the proximal interphalangeal joint. Hand Surg. 2015;20(1):107–14.
33. Waris E, Alanen V. Percutaneous, intramedullary fracture reduction and extension block pinning for dorsal proximal interphalangeal fracture-dislocations. J Hand Surg Am. 2010;35(12):2046–52.
34. Mangelson JJ, Stern P, Abzeg JM, Chang J, Osterman AL. Complications following dislocations of the proximal interphalangeal joint. J Bone Joint Surg Am. 2013;95:11326–32.
35. O'Rourke SK, Gaur S, Barton NJ. Long-term outcome of articular fractures of the phalange: an eleven year follow-up. J Hand Surg Br. 1989;14:183–93.
36. Blazar PE, Steinberg DR. Fractures of the proximal interphalangeal joint. J Am Acad Orthop Surg. 2000;8(6):383–90.

Chapter 10
Hemi-hamate Arthroplasty

Agnes Z. Dardas and Ryan P. Calfee

Abstract Hemi-hamate arthroplasty offers a unique reconstructive option for dorsal fracture-dislocations of the proximal interphalangeal joint. The distal articular surface of the hamate has a central ridge that is shaped similarly to that of the proximal articular surface of the middle phalanx making it an ideal osteochondral donor site. Hemi-hamate arthroplasty is indicated in both acute and chronic injuries that are not amenable to primary fracture fixation. Use of this osteochondral autograft requires an intact dorsal cortex with dorsal articular surface for fixation. The hamate graft is inset to recreate the volar buttress of the middle phalanx to prevent recurrent dorsal subluxation at the proximal interphalangeal joint. Although the outcomes after hemi-hamate arthroplasty are mostly reported in small case series, the outcomes of hemi-hamate arthroplasty are often very satisfactory. Reasonably good motion is to be expected, with flexion at the affected proximal interphalangeal joint approaching 90°, although a mild loss of terminal extension is common.

A.Z. Dardas, B.A. • R.P. Calfee, M.D., M.Sc. (✉)
Department of Orthopaedic Surgery, Washington
University School of Medicine, Campus Box 8233,
660 South Euclid Avenue, St. Louis, MO 63110, USA
e-mail: calfeer@wudosis.wustl.edu

© Springer International Publishing Switzerland 2016
J.E. Adams (ed.), *PIP Joint Fracture Dislocations*,
DOI 10.1007/978-3-319-28579-5_10

Keywords PIP joint • Interphalangeal • Fracture • Hemi-hamate
• Arthroplasty • Dislocation • Reconstruction • Autograft
• Subluxation • Salvage

Case

A 38-year-old female presented after injuring her dominant right ring finger. She thought that she had sprained her proximal interphalangeal (PIP) joint after an axial load injury from a volleyball 5 weeks prior. She initially treated the digit with ice and a nonsteroidal anti-inflammatory medication, but the finger was still stiff and painful. She denied prior injury to that digit. On physical exam, her right ring finger PIP joint was swollen. The finger had no malrotation but had a limited PIP arc of motion from 10° to 40°. The distal interphalangeal and metacarpal-phalangeal joints were nontender. Radiographs revealed a fracture of the volar articular surface of the middle phalanx at the PIP joint with dorsal subluxation of the PIP joint (Fig. 10.1). The dorsal articular surface of the middle phalanx was intact. The fracture was estimated to involve 50 % of the joint surface. At this point, the reconstructive option of a hemi-hamate arthroplasty was chosen. Because of the duration of time from injury to surgery and the presence of comminution, external fixation or open reduction internal fixation were unlikely to be successful. Therefore, the decision was made to proceed with hemi-hamate arthroplasty (Figs. 10.2, 10.3, 10.4, 10.5, 10.6, 10.7, and 10.8).

Rationale

PIP joint fracture-dislocations are complex injuries that even when treated appropriately can produce permanent stiffness and disability. Hastings' biomechanic study demonstrated that when ≥42 % of the palmar articular surface of the middle phalanx at the PIP joint is removed, joint subluxation consistently occurs [1]. Consistent

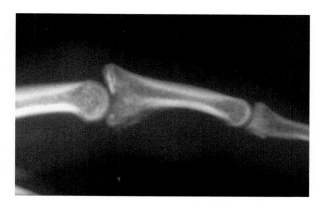

Fig. 10.1 Lateral radiograph of dorsal PIP fracture-dislocation involving 50 % of volar articular surface

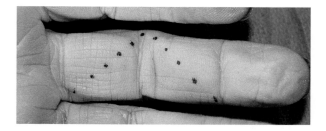

Fig. 10.2 V-shaped incision for hemi-hamate arthroplasty

with that early mechanical data, PIP joint fracture-dislocations are routinely classified into three types: "stable," involving less than 30 % of the volar articular base of the middle phalanx; "tenuous," involving 30–50 % of the base; and "unstable," involving greater than 50 % of the base.

Tenuous or unstable fractures frequently require ≥30–45° of PIP flexion to maintain a closed reduction. When excessive PIP flexion is required for a concentric reduction, surgical intervention is indicated to restore joint congruency. Although many treatment options exist, the hemi-hamate arthroplasty provides a reconstructive option for fractures

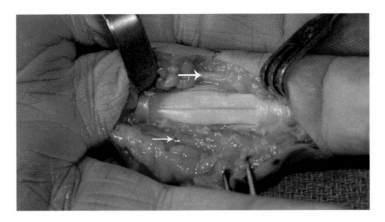

Fig. 10.3 Deep exposure with opening the flexor sheath between A2 and A4 with neurovascular bundles (*arrows*) dissected free

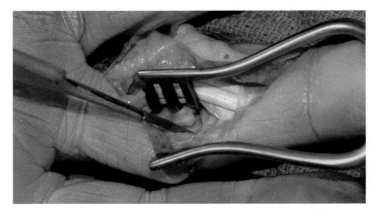

Fig. 10.4 Release of the accessory collateral ligament off the volar plate after release of the distal volar plate

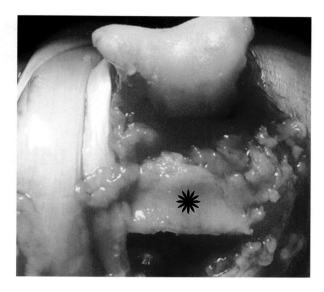

Fig. 10.5 Shotgunned PIP joint with articular surface of the middle phalanx (*) prepared to a level defect

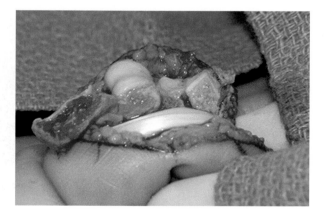

Fig. 10.6 Intraoperative lateral photograph confirming appropriate canting of hemi-hamate graft to restore concave articular surface

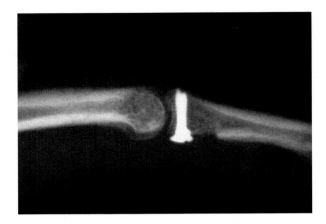

Fig. 10.7 Final lateral radiograph demonstrating congruent PIP joint

involving ≥50 % of the volar articular surface of the middle phalanx, comminuted fractures, and subacute or chronic injuries. Hemi-hamate arthroplasty (HHA) reconstructs the palmar lip of the proximal phalanx using the distal hamate articular surface (carpal-metacarpal joints). This bicondylar hamate surface articulates with the fourth and fifth metacarpals separated by a central ridge. This coronal plane-shape central ridge mirrors the bicondylar facet and central ridge of the proximal portion of the middle phalanx. In the sagittal plane, the phalangeal radius of curvature is only 45–61 % of the larger hamate, but canting the hamate graft during insertion allows effective restoration of a bony buttress to prevent PIP dorsal subluxation [2].

Indications and Contraindications

Hemi-hamate arthroplasty is a reconstructive option best suited for comminuted or chronic unstable fractures of the volar articular surface of the middle phalanx at the PIP joint. These fracture types often involve 50 % or more of the palmar articular surface or require 30° or more of flexion to maintain reduction [3]. An intact dorsal cortex is required to allow the relatively flat hamate restore

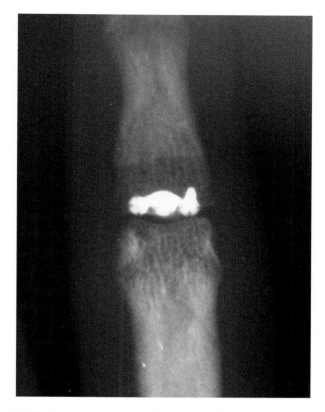

Fig. 10.8 Final anterior-posterior radiograph after hemi-hamate arthroplasty

the volar lip of the middle phalanx. While it is unknown how much dorsal articular surface needs to be intact, it is thought that fractures involving over 80 % of the joint surface may exceed the ability of the hamate to restore a concave articular surface due to increased risk of re-subluxation. In chronic irreducible injuries initially treated by other means, hemi-hamate arthroplasty can serve as a salvage procedure after failed external fixation, open reduction and internal fixation, or volar plate arthroplasty.

Contraindications to this surgical option include patients unable to comply with postoperative physical therapy, patients with preexisting degenerative arthritis of the affected PIP joint, and patients with pilon fractures involving 100 % of the articular surface. Hemi-hamate arthroplasty is not performed if the fracture is amenable to primary fixation of the fracture.

Surgical Technique

The surgical technique of hemi-hamate arthroplasty has been well documented since first described by Dr. Hastings in 1999 at the Annual Meeting of the American Society for Surgery of the Hand. A palmar Bruner-style "V" incision is centered at the PIP joint and extends from the distal interphalangeal joint flexion crease to the proximal digital crease (Fig. 10.2). The neurovascular bundles are identified and dissected from surrounding supportive tissues to prevent stretch injury when the PIP joint is hyperextended. The flexor tendon sheath is opened between the A2 and A4 pulleys (Fig. 10.3). The flexor tendons are retracted to either side, and the palmar plate of the PIP joint is retracted proximally after incising its distal insertion along with its radial and ulnar attachments to the accessory collateral ligaments (Fig. 10.4). The radial and ulnar collateral ligaments are released from their origins on the proximal phalanx, and the joint is hyperextended or "shotgunned" open. Once the joint is shotgunned, extensor tenolysis is performed to free the tendon from the proximal phalanx in chronic fracture-dislocations [4]. The articular surface of the middle phalanx is inspected, the fracture fragments are excised, and the site is prepared to accept the hemi-hamate graft. The articular surface is prepared to have a level surface of remaining dorsal cortex (Fig. 10.5), and radial and ulnar edges at the articular surface are preserved if possible to optimize subsequent graft fit. The metaphyseal void in the middle phalanx is prepared to a flat base, and if possible, this base gets progressively more shallow distally to aid in canting the graft toward the articular surface. The defect is measured in all dimensions in anticipation of graft harvest.

Harvesting the hamate is performed through an incision overlying the ulnar carpometacarpal joints, exposing the distal articular surface of the hamate with the fourth and fifth metacarpals. Caution is taken to preserve the dorsal cutaneous branches of the ulnar nerve when dissecting through the subcutaneous tissues. The hemi-hamate graft is harvested with two longitudinal cuts centered on the distal articular ridge and a proximal transverse cut. The bony cuts can be made with an osteotome connecting Kirschner wire holes or using an oscillating saw. Remove a small portion of dorsal hamate cortex proximal to the intended graft aids in harvesting a rectangular as opposed to a more triangular graft. Once the graft is procured, the dorsal capsular tissues are reapproximated, and the skin of the donor site is closed.

Final contouring of the graft is performed to match the prepared bed of the middle phalanx. It is then provisionally anchored with a single fine Kirschner wire before definitive fixation to the intact dorsal cortex with 2–3 screws, generally 1.3 or 1.5 mm in diameter. It is helpful to confirm that the graft is canted enough to produce the necessary volar lip after placing the Kirschner wire but before screw placement (Fig. 10.6). The joint is reduced, stability and range of motion are evaluated, and fluoroscopy is performed to confirm concentric reduction of the joint in flexion and extension, as well as screw position and length. Since the articular cartilage of the hamate graft is thicker than that on the base of the middle phalanx, imaging may reveal a step-off in the subchondral bone at the graft-host junction despite visual inspection revealing matched articular surfaces (Figs. 10.7 and 10.8). The distal corners of the palmar plate are repaired, the flexor tendon sheath is either transposed beneath the tendons or excised, and the skin is closed in a primary fashion. The hand is placed in a bulky dressing with a padded splint on the operated finger maintaining the PIP joint in approximately 15–20° of flexion.

Alternative Techniques

In an effort to minimize the risks of nonunion, excessive bone loss, and iatrogenic phalangeal fracture at the recipient site while addressing the need for distal palmar tilt, Yang et al. proposed an alternative method of osteotomy during graft harvest. In this modified technique, the fourth and fifth carpometacarpal joints are forcefully subluxated volarly to expose the distal articular surface of the hamate. The harvest of the graft in the coronal plane is then begun at the distal articular surface and continued in the proximal direction in a slightly volar angle so that the height of the proximal portion of the graft is higher than the height of the distal articular side. When placed in the straight bed of the recipient site, the graft is then naturally canted, thereby recreating the narrower cup-shaped articular surface of the middle phalangeal base [5].

Rozen et al. proposed harvesting a free vascularized hemi-hamate flap to reduce the risk of developing osteoarthritis from incomplete graft revascularization resulting in decrease in hyaline cartilage and subchondral necrosis. The vascular pedicle consists of efferent limbs arising from the intercarpal arch and a capsular vein that is re-anastomosed to the ulnar digital artery of the finger and a volar digital vein, respectively. Screw placement is modified to placement lateral to the periosteal attachments of the flap in order to preserve the periosteal supply [6]. Studies comparing the long-term outcomes of non-vascularized to vascularized hemi-hamate arthroplasties have yet to be published in order to determine if this truly aids in cartilage preservation, but the early postoperative course has been reported to be uneventful in terms of recipient and donor site morbidity.

Rehabilitation

Early hemi-hamate arthroplasty rehabilitation focuses on edema control, scar management, and early active motion with extension block splinting preventing 10–20° of terminal extension at the PIP joint for the first 4–6 weeks. Unrestricted heavy use of the hand for sports and similar activities is not recommended until radiographic demonstration of incorporation of the bone graft [7]. Mobilization of the DIP and MCP joints are encouraged throughout the process.

Outcomes

Hemi-hamate arthroplasty appears to reliably reduce pain, produce a functional PIP arc of motion, and prevent substantial upper extremity disability in both acute and chronic injuries (Table 10.1).

Table 10.1 Case series reporting hemi-hamate arthroplasty outcomes

Authors (year)	N	Joint involvement [min]	Time to surgery [range]	Mean follow-up months [min]	Final mean PIP Arc	% Contralateral grip strength	Mean residual pain	Mean DASH	Complications and revisions
Williams et al. (2003) [3]	13	60 % [40]	45 days [2–175]	16 [6]	85°	80 %	VAS: 1.3	–	Pain with overuse or cold temperatures: 6 Stiffness: 2 Recurrent dorsal subluxation: 2 Ulnar collapse, no graft resorption: 1

(continued)

Table 10.1 (continued)

Authors (year)	N	Joint involvement [min]	Time to surgery [range]	Mean follow-up months [min]	Final mean PIP Arc	% Contralateral grip strength	Mean residual pain	Mean DASH	Complications and revisions
Calfee et al. (2009)[a] [4]	22	63 % [50]	Acute <6 weeks; chronic >9 weeks	54 [12]	70°	95 %	VAS: 1.4 (acute 0.7, chronic 2.5)	5 (acute, 2; chronic, 9)	Aching with cold temperatures: 10 Flexor pulley insufficiency: 1 Severe flexion contracture (80°): 1 Silicone arthroplasty: 1
Afendras et al. (2010) [9]	8	61 % [52]	22 days [4–70]	60 [48]	67°	91 %	VAS (0–100), rest: 10 (0–70) mm VAS, activity: 17 (0–90) mm	Quick DASH: 19	Advanced arthritis: 2 Mild arthritis: 2 Flexor tenolysis: 1

Korambayil et al. (2011) [12]	5	60 % [50]	32 days [14–90]	22 [7]	94°	–	–	–	None
Lindenblatt et al. (2013) [13]	10	60 % [50]	93 days [0–371]	9 [3]	71°	95 %			Arthrolysis of the PIPJ: 2 Screw shortening: 2 Donor site neurolysis: 1
Yang et al. (2014) [5]	11	58 % [50]	4 days [2–7]	38 [34]	85°	94.5 %	VAS, rest: 0.27 cm VAS, activity: 1.2 cm	4.8	Radiographic signs of graft absorption: 1 Tenderness at donor site: 1 Mild arthritis: 1 Screw removal: 1

[a]Some patients also reported in series by Williams et al.

Most series report high patient satisfaction with a minority of surgical failures [8, 9]. Neither pain nor objective measures of function have been associated with percentage of joint surface involvement [4]. However, chronic reconstructions have been associated with increased VAS pain ratings and diminished grip strength as compared to acute reconstructions performed within 6 weeks of injury (Table 10.1) [4]. Radiographic signs of graft absorption [4], residual flexion contracture [4, 10], and mild recurrent dorsal subluxation [8] have all been noted but not clearly correlated with functional deficits or increased pain. Development of mild to severe osteoarthritis has also frequently been observed [4, 5, 9] and continues to remain a concern as patients are often relatively young, and published follow-up thus far has been limited to 7 years at most.

Few complications regarding donor site morbidity have been cited and include two cases of tenderness [5, 11] and one case of neuropathic pain secondary to tethering of the dorsal cutaneous branch of the ulnar nerve that improved after subsequent neurolysis [10]. Carpal-metacarpal joint instability has not been reported.

Salvage Options

Since hemi-hamate arthroplasty is reserved for unstable and comminuted PIP joint articular surface fractures, salvage options after a failed procedure are limited. Clinically, failure is typically manifest by persistent pain, unacceptable deformity, or lost motion. Unless a modifiable technical complication is encountered, a salvage silicone arthroplasty, arthrodesis, or amputation is considered.

References

1. Hastings H, II, Hamlet WP. Critical assessment of PIP joint stability after palmar lip fracture dislocations. 56th Annual Meeting of the American Society for Surgery of the Hand 2001; Baltimore, MD:(Abstract).
2. Capo JT, Hastings H, Choung E, Kinchelow T, Rossy W, Steinberg B. Hemicondylar hamate replacement arthroplasty for proximal interpha-

langeal joint fracture dislocations: an assessment of graft suitability. J Hand Surg Am. 2008;33(5):733–9.

3. Williams RMM, Hastings H, Kiefhaber TR. PIP fracture/dislocation treatment technique: use of a hemi-hamate resurfacing arthroplasty. Tech Hand Up Extrem Surg. 2002;6(4):185–92.

4. Calfee RP, Kiefhaber TR, Sommerkamp TG, Stern PJ. Hemi-hamate arthroplasty provides functional reconstruction of acute and chronic proximal interphalangeal fracture-dislocations. J Hand Surg Am. 2009;34(7): 1232–41.

5. Yang DS, Lee SK, Kim KJ, Choy WS. Modified hemi-hamate arthroplasty technique for treatment of acute proximal interphalangeal joint fracture-dislocations. Ann Plast Surg. 2014;72(4):411–6.

6. Rozen WM, Niumsawatt V, Leong JC, Ek EW. The vascular basis of the hemi-hamate osteochondral free flap. Part 2: Surgical anatomy and clinical application. Surg Radiol Anat. 2013;35(7):595–608.

7. McAuliffe JA. Hemi-hamate autograft for the treatment of unstable dorsal fracture dislocation of the proximal interphalangeal joint. J Hand Surg Am. 2009;34(10):1890–4.

8. Williams RMM, Kiefhaber TR, Sommerkamp TG, Stern PJ. Proximal interphalangeal fracture/dislocations using a hemi-hamate autograft. J Hand Surg Am. 2003;28A(5):856–65.

9. Afendras G, Abramo A, Mrkonjic A, Geijer M, Kopylov P, Ta M. Hemi-hamate osteochondral transplantation in proximal interphalangeal dorsal fracture dislocations: a minimum 4 year follow-up in eight patients. J Hand Surg Eur Vol. 2010;35E(8):627–31.

10. Lindenblatt N, Biraima A, Tami I, Giovanoli P, Calcagni M. Hemi-hamate autograft arthroplasty for acute and chronic PIP joint fracture dislocations. Handchir Mikrochir Plast Chir. 2013;45(1):13–9.

11. Rozen WM, Niumsawatt V, Ross R, Leong JC, Ek EW. The vascular basis of the hemi-hamate osteochondral free flap. Part 1: Vascular anatomy and clinical correlation. Surg Radiol Anat. 2013;35(7):585–94.

12. Korambayil PM, Francis A. Hemi-hamate arthroplasty for pilon fractures of finger. Indian J Plast Surg. 2015;44(3):458–66.

13. Bigorre N, Rabarin F, Jeudy J, Césari B. [Treatment for a chronic proximal interphalangeal fracture-dislocation with hemi-hamate arthroplasty]. Chir Main. 2014;33(2):148–52.

Chapter 11
Condylar Replacement Arthroplasty and Other PIP Autografts

John R. Lien and T. Greg Sommerkamp

Abstract Proximal interphalangeal (PIP) joint injuries with associated osteochondral defects are a challenging problem. Without restoration of a concentrically reduced PIP joint, post-traumatic articular degenerative changes will develop. The indications for hemihamate replacement arthroplasty (HHRA) are limited to volar defects of the middle phalanx base with an intact dorsal cortex and at least 10–20 % of the dorsal articular surface remaining on the base of the middle phalanx. Other osteoarticular PIP joint injuries include middle phalanx base sagittal defects, proximal phalanx unicondylar defects, combined proximal and middle phalangeal osteochondral defects from open injury, and isolated focal osteochondral defects. The goal of this chapter is to provide an overview of autograft options (other than HHRA) for PIP joint osteochondral defects, with a clinical vignette demonstrating reconstruction of a unicondylar injury of the proximal phalanx.

J.R. Lien, M.D.
Department of Orthopaedic Surgery, University of Michigan Health Systems, 2098 South Main Street, Ann Arbor, MI 48103, USA
e-mail: jlien@med.umich.edu

T.G. Sommerkamp, M.D. (✉)
Tri Health- Hand Surgery Specialists, Inc., 545 Centre View Blvd, Crestview Hills, KY 41017, USA
e-mail: thomas_sommerkamp@trihealth.com

© Springer International Publishing Switzerland 2016   141
J.E. Adams (ed.), *PIP Joint Fracture Dislocations*,
DOI 10.1007/978-3-319-28579-5_11

Keywords   Proximal interphalangeal joint • Osteochondral arthroplasty • Proximal phalanx condyle fracture • Condylar replacement
arthroplasty

Introduction

Proximal interphalangeal (PIP) joint injuries with associated osteochondral defects are a challenging problem. These injuries may
present acutely, with severely comminuted and/or open articular
fractures, as well as in a subacute setting with malunited or
resorbed periarticular fractures. Pain, swelling, limited range of
motion (ROM), angular deformity, and rotational deformity may be
appreciated. Without restoration of a concentrically reduced PIP
joint, posttraumatic articular degenerative changes will develop.

The hemihamate replacement arthroplasty (HHRA) is an effective
tool in the management of severe dorsal PIP fracture dislocations.
However, the indications for HHRA are limited to volar defects of the
middle phalanx base with an intact dorsal cortex and at least 10–20 %
of the dorsal articular surface remaining on the base of the middle
phalanx. Other osteoarticular PIP joint injuries include middle phalanx base sagittal defects, proximal phalanx unicondylar defects,
combined proximal and middle phalangeal osteochondral defects
from open injury, and isolated focal osteochondral defects.

The goal of this chapter is to provide an overview of autograft
options (other than HHRA) for PIP joint osteochondral defects, with
a clinical vignette demonstrating reconstruction of a unicondylar
injury of the proximal phalanx.

Management Options

Prior to considering autograft reconstruction, if the fracture is relatively acute and the fragments are of reasonable size, one must
consider open reduction and internal fixation or other means of
maintaining a stable reduction. In the setting of malunion, osteotomy

with internal fixation is an option if the articular surface is preserved and there is adequate bone stock. Other tools include implant arthroplasty and joint arthrodesis. Patient factors such as activity level, age, and comorbidities are important in determining management. The ideal candidate for autograft reconstruction is a young, active patient who wishes to preserve joint motion.

Many methods of autograft reconstruction have been described, but most outcome data are limited to small case series.

Total Joint Transfer

Vascularized second toe joint transfer is useful in situations with proximal and distal articular loss, as well as composite dorsal tissue deficit [1]. Additionally, growth potential of the epiphysis may be maintained in the pediatric patient. However, it is a technically demanding microsurgical procedure not without morbidity. Additionally, joint flexion contractures and extensor lag with a limited arc of motion are common outcomes with this procedure.

Vascularized homodigital and heterodigital joint transfer may be used in traumatic situations as "spare part" surgery. As with toe joint transfer, this technique is useful in the setting of total joint destruction as well as composite tissue loss. Since the donor finger is nonsalvageable due to other injuries, these procedures carry no additional morbidity. Both island and free joint transfer, either from the PIP or distal interphalangeal (DIP) joint, have been described [2].

Partial Articular Reconstruction

Osteochondral autograft transfer utilizes osteochondral plugs from either hamate or knee donor [3, 4]. This can be performed on either the proximal phalanx or middle phalanx articular surface and may be useful in patients with focal osteoarticular defects. However, in order to maintain press-fit fixation, an intact rim of articular cartilage or cortex is necessary.

Nonvascularized hemi-toe autograft may be used to reconstruct the proximal phalanx condyle [5] as well as full-thickness sagittal defects (involving volar and dorsal cortices) in the middle phalanx base [6]. Morphometric studies show the third toe proximal phalanx distal articular surface and the medial base of the toe middle phalanx most closely approximate the PIP recipient site [7].

Costal perichondrial resurfacing may produce a fibrocartilage articular surface but cannot compensate for bony defects and concomitant angular deformity. Additionally, problems with substantial joint stiffness are recognized in follow-up [8]. Chondroperichondrial grafting has also been described, but is also reserved for salvage arthroplasty [9]. Costal cartilage autograft reconstruction provides a structural support to correct bone loss and produces hyaline cartilage [10] but also has problems with stiffness, with one series reporting a 33° average arc of motion [11]. Potential problems with this donor area during harvest, though unlikely, can be substantial.

Portions of the second and third carpometacarpal (CMC) joints can be harvested for nonvascularized osteoarticular autograft and for reconstruction of proximal phalanx condyle (capitate donor) as well as middle phalanx base (metacarpal base donor) defects [12]. In addition, a pedicled osteoarticular distal capitate flap, based on the second or third dorsal metacarpal artery, can be used for reconstruction of a unicondylar proximal phalanx defect. A theoretical advantage is the vascularity of the graft, which may help with incorporation and viability of the chondrocytes. While no avascular necrosis (AVN) was observed, 3 of 15 patients who underwent flap autograft had PIP joint space narrowing at follow-up [13].

The fourth and fifth metacarpal (MC) bases have been morphometrically compared as potential donor sites for proximal phalanx condylar replacement arthroplasty [14]. The small MC base has a radius of curvature (ROC) that more closely resembles that of the phalangeal condyles, and this correlation between donor and recipient appears to remain constant despite variations in hand size. A clinical series demonstrated reconstruction using fifth MC base osteoarticular autograft, with acceptable results at an average of 4.8-year follow-up [15].

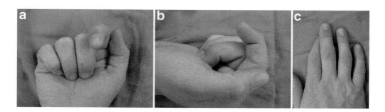

Fig. 11.1 Preoperative physical exam findings: ulnar deviation and supination deformity and limited PIP range of motion

Clinical Vignette

Clinical Problem

A 21-year-old right-hand dominant male sustained a right index proximal phalanx comminuted ulnar condyle fracture. He was initially treated with "buddy taping" of the index finger to the adjacent long finger by the initial treating orthopedic surgeon. He presented 6 months later with stiffness, loss of motion, PIP pain, and angular/rotational deformity at the PIP joint.

Examination

Active ROM upon presentation was MP +20–85°, PIP 26–56°, and DIP 4–65°. Passive ROM was MP +25–90°, PIP 20–60°, and DIP 0–70°. Deformities in ulnar deviation (20°) and supination (10°) at the level of the PIP joint were also noted (Fig. 11.1). Radiographs revealed an ulnar condyle malunion with loss of condylar height, bone resorption, and a bony flexion block deformity (Fig. 11.2a).

Procedure: Condylar Replacement Arthroplasty (CRA)

We recommended CRA using the base of the small metacarpal as the source of the osteochondral autograft. Rationale for this graft includes minimal donor-site morbidity, technical practicality, and relationship to normal condylar morphology [14].

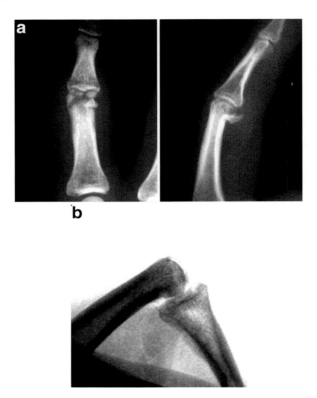

Fig. 11.2 Radiographic views of the index finger PIP joint preoperative (**a**) and intraoperative (**b**). (**a**) The preoperative films demonstrate a proximal phalangeal ulnar condyle malunion. (**b**) Intraoperative films show improved flexion following excision of the deformed ulnar condyle

The index ulnar condyle was exposed through an ulnar mid-axial approach. The transverse retinacular ligament was sharply divided just volar to the lateral band. The capsule was identified and a capsulotomy was performed. The ulnar collateral ligament (UCL) origin was subperiosteally dissected off the damaged ulnar condyle and saved for later UCL reconstruction. The PIP joint was then completely exposed by a modified "shotgun" exposure hinging the middle phalanx around the intact radial collateral ligament. Upon exposure of

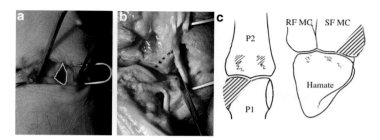

Fig. 11.3 (**a, b**) Harvest of small metacarpal base (cadaver on right), (**c**) illustration of small finger metacarpal base donor site and proximal phalanx recipient site

the PIP joint, the degenerative changes over the ulnar condyle were noted. In addition, the bony block to flexion was identified and removed. Intraoperative flexion improved from 60° to 90° (Fig. 11.2b), yet ulnar deviation and supination deformity persisted. The comminuted, malunited ulnar condyle was unreconstructable and removed through an oblique osteotomy which was performed in the anterior-posterior plane. An oblique osteotomy provided a maximum amount of cancellous bone surface to support and secure the graft and augment rapid revascularization.

Next, the small finger CMC joint was exposed through a transverse incision approximately 2 cm in length. The CMC joint was exposed between the extensor carpi ulnaris and extensor digiti quinti tendons. A capsulotomy was performed making sure to remove the ulnar portion of the CMC ligament from the hamate and leaving a portion of it attached to the ulnar base of the small MC to be used for later reattachment to the ulnar collateral ligament of the PIP joint. The condylar defect was measured, and the appropriate amount of graft was harvested from the ulnar aspect of the small finger MC base (Fig. 11.3a–c). The extensor carpi ulnaris tendinous insertion was partially reflected distally from its attachment when necessary to obtain adequate graft material (Fig. 11.3b). The entire dorsal-volar dimension was included in the graft, whereas only the necessary radial-ulnar dimension was obtained. Once the graft was harvested, the remaining CMC joint was tested for stability directly by grasping the remaining intact base and attempting to dislocate the joint and

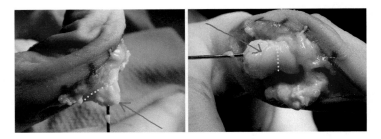

Fig. 11.4 Provisional fixation of condylar replacement autograft. *Red arrow* depicts CRA graft; *dashed yellow lines* depict osteotomy site

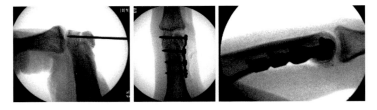

Fig. 11.5 Provisional then definitive fixation of CRA graft with A.O./Synthes 1.5 mm minicondylar plate

indirectly by flexing and extending the metacarpal and observing for subluxation, and none was present.

Following harvest, the graft was appropriately positioned in the proximal phalangeal defect and provisionally fixed with a Kirschner wire (Fig. 11.4). Definitive fixation was then performed with a 1.5 mm A.O./Synthes minicondylar plate over the provisional wire. Intraoperative radiographs revealed excellent alignment and position, and the wire was replaced with a 1.5 mm lag screw placed across the CRA graft into the radial condyle (Fig. 11.5). It is important to position the graft such that any excess in the anterior-posterior dimension is directed dorsally. Thus, if any dorsal trimming of excess graft is required, the volar articular contour of the graft is preserved, thereby allowing maximal flexion. Once positioned and trimmed, the PIP joint was reduced. The ulnar collateral ligament was then repaired to the CMC ligament remaining on the graft. Stability and ROM were tested.

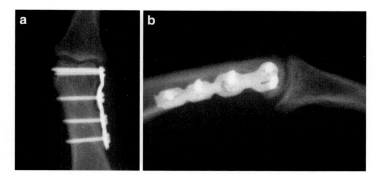

Fig. 11.6 Postoperative films demonstrate that the graft has incorporated into the host bone without evidence of AVN and maintenance of the joint space at 2 years

Postoperatively, immobilization consisted of a volar positioning splint. Full active ROM was initiated 48 h after surgery, with active-assisted ROM starting 1 week postoperatively. The index finger was well aligned with improved PIP AROM (10–90°) achieved by 10 weeks which was slightly reduced at 36 months (25–90°). Representative radiographs at 24 months postoperatively revealed complete incorporation of the graft with preservation of joint space and no evidence of avascular necrosis (Fig. 11.6). At 36 months, the patient did complain of hardware tenderness from the prominent "shoulder" of the 1.5 mm minicondylar implant and underwent successful hardware removal, tenolysis, and capsulectomy. A small cartilage punch biopsy of the peripheral articular rim of the CRA autograft obtained at the time of the hardware removal revealed viable hyaline cartilage with numerous chondrocytes (Fig. 11.7). The final active ROM at 48 months was PIP 15–95° and DIP 0–65°. X-rays at 48 months revealed the CRA graft to be well incorporated and revascularized without any plain radiographic changes of AVN or post-traumatic osteoarthritis (Fig. 11.8). There was no instability or arthrosis at the donor site.

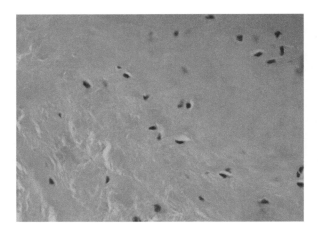

Fig. 11.7 Photomicrograph of a biopsy obtained from the most peripheral rim of the CRA graft demonstrating viable chondrocytes in the peripheral fibrocartilage

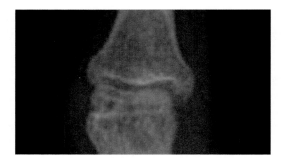

Fig. 11.8 Radiograph of PIP joint at 4 years post-op, after hardware removal. Note ulnar condyle with normal radiodensity and no sign of late segmental collapse, with well-preserved joint space

Discussion

As part of our earlier lab research [14], the base of the small and ring finger metacarpals was morphometrically assessed as potential donors to replace one of the condyles of the proximal phalanx. Of the two donor grafts investigated, only the small MC base demonstrated adequate graft material to resurface all dimensions of the phalangeal condyles. Both potential donors demonstrated adequate graft in the anterior-posterior and dorsal radial-ulnar dimensions. When assessing volar width, however, only the small MC base had more osteocartilaginous stock than the recipient condyles to assure room for adjustments. The ring MC base, on the other hand, had just enough material, which provides minimal room for error in making adjustments in the volar dimension. In addition, since all of the volar surface must be harvested, ring CMC instability is of concern. These would not be concerns for the small MC base as there is adequate material in all dimensions.

Although the ring MC base has enough stock to reconstruct some of the condyles, another confounding variable is its large radius of curvature that makes it less suited for condylar reconstruction. The small MC base, on the other hand, has a lower radius of curvature that more closely approximates that of the phalangeal condyles. In addition, regression analysis demonstrated that the relationship in ROC between donor and recipient is stronger if the small MC base is used as the donor. Thus, the surgeon can be confident that the correlation between donor and recipient will remain a constant, despite variation in hand size.

Both the ulnar as well as the radial base of the small metacarpal can be utilized; however, the ulnar base is simpler to harvest. The radial base is bordered by the ring MC base and thus makes it more difficult to harvest. Although, the ulnar base was used to resurface an ulnar condyle in both our cadaveric preparations and in the case example, the same ulnar base can also be used to resurface the radial condyle after being rotated appropriately.

In the ulnar two digits, the radial condyle is more frequently fractured than the ulnar condyle [16]. The opposite occurs for the radial two digits, i.e., the ulnar condyle is more frequently fractured than the radial condyle. Interestingly, the condyles that are frequently fractured also happen to be the larger condyles by measurements obtained in our prior studies [14]. Given that the small finger MC graft has a larger radius of curvature than any of the native condyles, it is optimal that the frequently injured condyles are of larger size. This makes those condyles that are frequently damaged a better match for the small MC donor CRA graft.

Development of osteoarthritis at the donor site is a legitimate concern following harvest. The data in the present study demonstrates that CMC stability is not altered by graft harvest. Therefore, given that the CMC joint is stable following harvest, the likelihood of developing OA is less likely than if instability was encountered. In the study by Williams et al., no donor-site morbidity was encountered in their series of hemihamate harvests for the hamate hemiarticular replacement arthroplasty (HHRA) [17] as well as in a 10-year follow-up study by Calfee et al. [18].

Another concern following autograft reconstruction is the viability of the osteochondral graft. Williams et al. demonstrated graft survivability in all patients treated with distal hamate osteochondral grafting for dorsal PIP fracture dislocations [17]. This is consistent with studies examining unicondylar grafts [19, 20]. However, grafts used to reconstruct both condyles have been met with less success [12]. The case example in this report demonstrated survivability of the unicondylar graft at latest follow-up of 48 months with normal radiographic appearance (Fig. 11.8) and viable chondrocytes on histology (Fig. 11.7).

Our studies have demonstrated that the base of the small MC is of appropriate dimensions to be suited for osteochondral donor material to resurface the proximal phalangeal condyles. In addition, the graft is simple to harvest and results in minimal morbidity with respect to CMC stability. Of the previously discussed autografts for condylar reconstruction, we believe that the base of the small MC is the optimal donor material.

The presumptive indications for condylar replacement arthroplasty using the ulnar base of the small MC include both acute and chronic conditions. In the acute situation, it is conceivable that CRA can be used for severely comminuted condyle fractures with an unreconstructable articular surface or complete condylar destruction by power saws. It can also be used in the chronic situation where malunion of the condyle fracture is associated with posttraumatic osteoarthritis where the middle phalanx base is minimally involved.

References

1. Tsubokawa N, Yoshizu T, Maki Y. Long-term results of free vascularized second toe joint transfers to finger proximal interphalangeal joints. J Hand Surg Am. 2003;28A:443–7. doi:10.1053/jhsu.2003.50087.

2. Foucher G, Lenoble E, Smith D. Free and island vascularized joint transfer for proximal interphalangeal reconstruction: a series of 27 cases. J Hand Surg Am. 1994;19A:8–16. doi:10.1016/0363-5023(94)90217-8.

3. Ozyurekoglu T. Multiple osteochondral autograft transfer to the proximal interphalangeal joint: case report. J Hand Surg Am. 2010;35A:931–5. doi:10.1016/j.jhsa.2010.02.034.

4. Yamagami N, Yamamoto S, Tsujimoto Y, Uchio Y. Osteochondral autograft transplantation for malunited intra-articular fracture of the proximal interphalangeal joint: a case report. Arch Orthop Trauma Surg. 2013;133:135–9. doi:10.1007/s00402-012-1622-4.

5. Gaul JS. Articular fractures of the proximal interphalangeal joint with missing elements: repair with partial toe joint osteochondral autografts. J Hand Surg Am. 1999;24A:78–85. doi:10.1053/jhsu.1999.jhsu24a0078.

6. Pirani AA, Rao A, Sharma S. Traumatic proximal interphalangeal joint reconstruction with an autologous hemi-toe osteochondral graft: case report. J Hand Surg Am. 2013;38A:1320–3. doi:10.1016/j.jhsa.2013.03.045.

7. Hendry JM, Mainprize J, McMillan C, Binhammer P. Structural comparison of the finger proximal interphalangeal joint surfaces and those of the third toe: suitability for joint reconstruction. J Hand Surg Am. 2011; 36A:1022–7. doi:10.1016/j.jhsa.2011.01.047.

8. Seradge H, Kutz JA, Kleinert HE, Lister GD, Wolff TW, Atasoy E. Perichondrial resurfacing arthroplasty in the hand. J Hand Surg Am. 1984;9A:880–6. doi:10.1016/S0363-5023(84)80072-6.

9. Takayama S, Nakao Y, Horiuchi Y, Itoh Y. Arthroplasty of MP and PIP joints using a chondroperichondrial graft. Tech Hand Up Extrem Surg. 1998;2(2):115–8. doi:10.1097/00130911-199806000-00005.

10. Sato K, Sasaki T, Nakamura T, Toyama Y, Ikegami H. Clinical outcome and histologic findings of costal osteochondral grafts for cartilage defects in finger joints. J Hand Surg Am. 2008;33A:511–5. doi:10.1016/j.jhsa.2008.01.003.

11. Zappaterra T, Obert L, Pauchot J, Lepage D, Rochet S, Gallinet D, et al. Post-traumatic reconstruction of digital joints by costal cartilage grafting: a preliminary prospective study. Chir Main. 2010;29:294–300. doi:10.1016/j.main.2010.07.003.

12. Ishida O, Ikuta Y, Kuroki H. Ipsilateral osteochondral grafting for finger joint repair. J Hand Surg Am. 1994;19A:372–7. doi:10.1016/0363-5023(94)90048-5.

13. Zhang X, Fang X, Shao X, Wen S, Zhu H, Ren C. Osteoarticular pedicle flap from the capitate to reconstruct traumatic defects in the head of the proximal phalanx. J Hand Surg Am. 2012;37A:1780–90. doi:10.1016/j.jhsa.2012.05.004.

154 J.R. Lien and T.G. Sommerkamp

14. Hernandez JD, Sommerkamp TG. Morphometric analysis of potential osteochondral autografts for resurfacing unicondylar defects of the proximal phalanx in PIP joint injuries. J Hand Surg Am. 2010;35A:604–10. doi:10.1016/j.jhsa.2009.12.041.
15. Cavadas PC, Landin L, Thione A. Reconstruction of the condyles of the proximal phalanx with osteochondral grafts from the ulnar base of the little finger metacarpal. J Hand Surg Am. 2010;35A:1275–81. doi:10.1016/j.jhsa.2010.04.013.
16. Weiss AP, Hastings H. Distal unicondylar fractures of the proximal phalanx. J Hand Surg Am. 1993;18A:594–9. doi:10.1016/0363-5023(93)90297-G.
17. Williams RM, Kiefhaber TR, Sommerkamp TG, Stern PJ. Treatment of unstable dorsal proximal interphalangeal fracture/dislocations using a hemi-hamate autograft. J Hand Surg Am. 2003;28A:856–65. doi:10.1016/S0363-5023(03)00304-6.
18. Calfee RP, Kiefhaber TR, Sommerkamp TG, Stern PJ. Hemi-hamate arthroplasty provides functional reconstruction of acute and chronic proximal interphalangeal fracture-dislocations. J Hand Surg Am. 2009;34A:1232–41. doi:10.1016/j.jhsa.2009.04.027.
19. Bury TF, Stassen LP, van der Werken C. Repair of the proximal interphalangeal joint with a homograft. J Hand Surg Am. 1989;14A:657–8. doi:10.1016/0363-5023(89)90185-8.
20. Hasegawa T, Yamano Y. Arthroplasty of the proximal interphalangeal joint using costal cartilage grafts. J Hand Surg Br. 1992;17B:583–5. doi:10.1016/S0266-7681(05)80248-7.

Chapter 12
Joint Replacement Arthroplasty: Is It Ever Indicated in PIP Joint Fracture-Dislocations?

H.L. Baltzer and Steven L. Moran

Abstract Reconstruction of the proximal interphalangeal (PIP) joint in the setting of post-traumatic joint arthritis is a challenging problem. When there is little range of motion preoperatively within the PIP joint, arthrodesis can be performed. Amputation can be offered in the setting of a stiff painful finger, but is generally not the first-line treatment and is rather a salvage procedure in the setting of a failed joint reconstruction. In patients wishing to maintain some range of joint motion and avoid fusion, PIP joint reconstruction can be performed with a variety of techniques including vascularized toe joint transfer, autologous non-vascularized hemihamate transfer, and replacement joint arthroplasty. A variety of materials have been tried for PIP joint arthroplasty including silicone [1], titanium [2], cobalt, chrome, and polyethylene [3]. While silicone PIP arthroplasty has the longest track record within

H.L. Baltzer, M.D., F.R.C.S.(C)
Division of Plastic and Reconstructive Surgery,
University of Toronto, Toronto, ON, Canada
e-mail: heather.baltzer@utoronto.ca

S.L. Moran, M.D. (✉)
Department of Plastic Surgery, Mayo Clinic Hospital,
Saint Mary's Campus, 200 First Street Southwest, Rochester, MN 55905, USA

Department of Orthopedic Surgery, Mayo Clinic Hospital,
Saint Mary's Campus, 200 First Street Southwest, Rochester, MN 55905, USA
e-mail: moran.steven@mayo.edu

© Springer International Publishing Switzerland 2016   155
J.E. Adams (ed.), *PIP Joint Fracture Dislocations*,
DOI 10.1007/978-3-319-28579-5_12

the United States, its nonanatomic design, limited durability, and limited stability make it a less than ideal choice for younger, more active patients. New options for PIP joint arthroplasty include the use of pyrocarbon. This chapter will examine the use of pyrocarbon arthroplasty following PIP trauma.

Keywords Arthroplasty • Proximal interphalangeal joint • Pyrocarbon • Hemiarthroplasty

Introduction

Reconstruction of the proximal interphalangeal (PIP) joint in the setting of post-traumatic joint arthritis is a challenging problem. When there is little range of motion preoperatively within the PIP joint, arthrodesis can be performed. Amputation can be offered in the setting of a stiff painful finger, but is generally not the first-line treatment and is rather a salvage procedure in the setting of a failed joint reconstruction. In patients wishing to maintain some range of joint motion and avoid fusion, PIP joint reconstruction can be performed with a variety of techniques including vascularized toe joint transfer, autologous non-vascularized hemi-hamate transfer, and replacement joint arthroplasty. A variety of materials have been tried for PIP joint arthroplasty including silicone [1], titanium [2], cobalt, chrome, and polyethylene [3]. While silicone PIP arthroplasty has the longest track record within the United States, its nonanatomic design, limited durability, and limited stability make it a less than ideal choice for younger, more active patients.

Other types of PIP arthroplasty have become popular in the United States and have included the use of PyroCarbon PIP joint arthroplasty. PyroCarbon implants were designed to function as unconstrained biologically inert anatomic implants for the replacement of the MCP joint in the late 1970s. Pyrolytic carbon is biologically compatible and has an elastic modulus similar to cortical bone, which presumably aids in dampening stresses at the bone prosthetic interface [4, 5]. The PyroCarbon implants are made of a graphite core coated with pyrolytic carbon, which is a coating material made by heating propane to

1300 °C [5]. The implant is used in a press-fit fashion without cement fixation. The non-cemented technique avoids the potential complications of cement use and facilitates easier revisions with significantly less bone stock compromise.

PyroCarbon (Ascension Orthopedics, Austin, TX) PIP implant arthroplasty was approved by the US Food and Drug Administration in 2002. The on-label use resurfaces both the head of the proximal phalanx and the base of the middle phalanx with a low-wear, chemically inert implant material. If only one joint surface is compromised in a post-traumatic setting, then a hemiarthroplasty may be indicated; however, this is off-label use of the PyroCarbon implants. In this chapter, a case of a total PIPJ arthroplasty and an off-label hemiarthroplasty will be presented and discussed.

Key considerations for using PyroCarbon implants in a post-traumatic setting include the integrity of the bone and overlying soft tissue. There must be some preservation of the collateral ligaments. In addition, there must be adequate bone stock to support the implant with a sufficient intramedullary space. Compromised soft tissue and evidence of active or chronic infection are contraindications to PyroCarbon arthroplasty [6]. During the preoperative discussion of the risks of PIP PyroCarbon arthroplasty, the surgeon should discuss the possibility of implant dislocation, implant subsidence, fracture, infection, and the potential need for PIP joint arthrodesis in the future if the joint replacement fails to provide stabile pain-free motion. Reports of revision surgery after post-traumatic PIPJ PyroCarbon arthroplasty can be as high as 33 % [7].

Literature reporting outcomes of post-traumatic PyroCarbon PIP joint arthroplasty are limited and retrospective. A recent systematic review comparing post-traumatic PIP joint arthroplasty using either vascularized toe joint transfer, silicone arthroplasty, or PyroCarbon arthroplasty found that the mean PIP joint active arcs of motion were 37.9°, 44.11°, and 43.11°, respectively [7]. The PyroCarbon data was taken from two small retrospective series which demonstrated no significant change in the PIP joint range of motion following surgery; however, postoperative grip and pinch strength increased significantly [8, 9].

In this chapter, we will present two cases of post-traumatic PyroCarbon arthroplasty, including an off-label use of the device as a hemiarthroplasty.

Case 1: PyroCarbon Arthroplasty Status Post-fracture-Dislocation of the PIP Joint

An 18-year-old male sustained a proximal phalanx condylar fracture of the right small finger 1 year prior to consultation with our team. At the time of the injury, initial management entailed closed reduction and percutaneous pinning of the fracture at an outside institution. Unfortunately, this was complicated by a pin-site infection that appeared to have involved the articular surface. Subsequent to this, he developed persistent swelling and pain over the small finger PIPJ and resultant painful, limited range of motion. He was otherwise healthy.

On physical examination, the affected right small finger had no evidence of ongoing infection. An early boutonniere deformity had developed, with an extension lag of 40° and active flexion of 65°. The remainder of the upper extremity examination was within normal limits. Baseline radiographs demonstrated malunion of the ulnar condyle of the proximal phalanx and advanced osteolysis of the joint surface with resultant post-traumatic degenerative osteoarthritis of the PIPJ (Fig. 12.1a–c). There was no remaining lucency to indicate an ongoing infective process, and bone scan was negative for osteomyelitis.

The patient was offered the options of placement of PyroCarbon PIP joint arthroplasty, arthrodesis, or amputation. Considering his age and desire to maintain motion in the PIP joint and the absence of persistent infection, the patient was deemed a good candidate for motion preserving surgery with arthroplasty.

This patient underwent a PyroCarbon arthroplasty of the small finger PIP joint (technique described in detail below). Four weeks postoperatively, the patient was assessed in follow-up, and a dislocation of the implant was discovered (Fig. 12.2a1–3), for which the patient was taken back to the operating room for a revision arthroplasty. The results following the revision are demonstrated in Fig. 12.2b1–3. At most recent follow-up (2 years postoperatively), the patient reported pain-free motion and satisfaction with his operative result. He reported that the joint was no longer a source of pain or concern for him. Physical examination revealed a 15° extension deficit at the PIP joint and active flexion of 55°

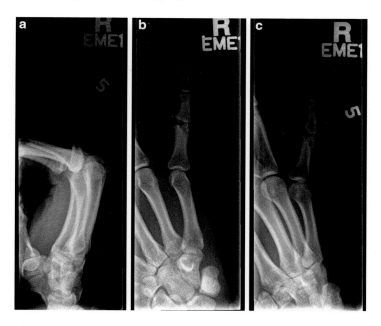

Fig. 12.1 Status post-unicondylar fracture of the small finger proximal phalanx, complicated by pin-tract infection with early hardware removal and resultant malunion of the proximal phalanx head. There is advanced osteolysis of the joint surface with post-traumatic degenerative osteoarthritis of the PIPJ

(Fig. 12.3a1, 2). He also had a 15° extension deficit at the DIP joint with active flexion of 15°. Range of motion was normal in the MCP joint. Radiographic assessment demonstrated good alignment with a small amount of implant subsidence (Fig. 12.3b1, 2).

Case 2: PIP Joint PyroCarbon Hemiarthroplasty

A 16-year-old male presenting 6 months status post-open reduction and internal fixation (ORIF) of a unicondylar fracture of the radial condyle of the proximal phalanx with concomitant

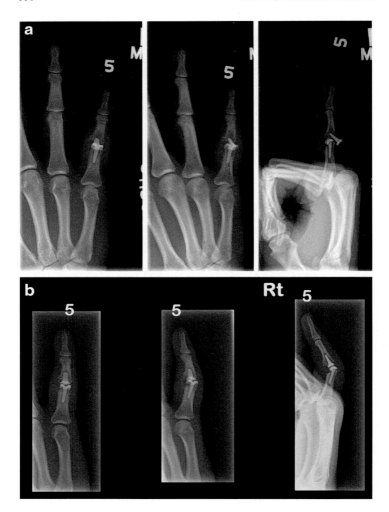

Fig. 12.2 (**a**) Four weeks post-PIPJ PyroCarbon arthroplasty. Patient presented with dislocation of implant requiring return to the operating room and revision of the arthroplasty. (**b**) Post-revision PIPJ arthroplasty with evidence of good alignment of the implant

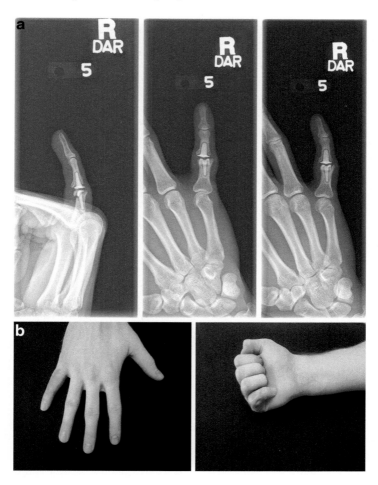

Fig. 12.3 Two years post-PIPJ PyroCarbon arthroplasty. (**a**) Patient has maintained painless range of motion and is satisfied with the result. (**b**) Radiographic assessment demonstrated good alignment with a small amount of implant subsidence at 2 years

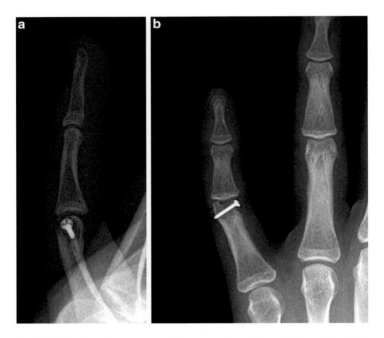

Fig. 12.4 Radiographs demonstrating resorption of the radial condyle of the proximal phalanx and incongruity of the proximal phalanx articular surface. There was prominence of the mini-screw into the articular surface radially. The middle phalanx articular surface appeared to be intact

dislocation of the left small finger PIP joint. The original injury occurred during a football game. An attempted open reduction and internal fixation was performed at an outside facility using mini-screw fixation. He subsequently developed painful, symptomatic arthritis and presented to our facility to discuss options for joint surface reconstruction. He was otherwise healthy. Physical examination demonstrated radial deviation at the PIP joint. The finger was maintained in an extended position with only 10° of active flexion that was extremely painful.

Radiographs demonstrated evidence of arthritis primarily affecting the head of the proximal phalanx (Fig. 12.4). The radial condyle had undergone significant resorption creating incongruity of the proximal phalanx articular surface and prominence of the mini-

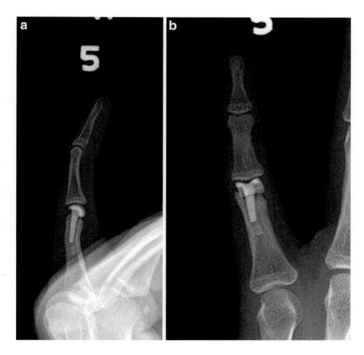

Fig. 12.5 Twelve months post-hemiarthroplasty of the small finger PIPJ with a PyroCarbon implant

screw into the articular surface radially. The middle phalanx articular surface appeared to be intact.

PyroCarbon hemiarthroplasty and a vascularized toe joint transfer were offered to the patient as reconstructive options. The patient elected to proceed with pyrolytic carbon implant hemiarthroplasty.

Postoperatively, the patient did well and began a short arc range of motion protocol. At last follow-up (18 months postoperatively), the patient has pain-free motion. Active ROM of the left small finger MCP, PIP, and DIP joints were 20–100°, 0–60°, and 0–70°, respectively. Radiographs demonstrate the implant positioned appropriately with no evidence of periprosthetic lucency (Fig. 12.5).

Surgical Technique: PyroCarbon PIP Joint Arthroplasty

General anesthesia, regional block, or local hand blocks are all appropriate forms of anesthesia for this procedure. We prefer the use of regional or local blocks. Tourniquet control is recommended.

Joint Exposure

A straight dorsal longitudinal incision approximately 2.5 cm in length is used to approach the PIP joint. In these cases, there was preexisting dorsal-ulnar scar from the previous surgeries that had been used. After identifying the extensor mechanism, full-thickness skin and subcutaneous tissue flaps should be elevated. We prefer an extensor-splitting approach to the joint; however, a Chamay technique could also be used (Fig. 12.6a, b). If an extensor-splitting approach is taken, a longitudinal incision is made over the PIPJ, and the central slip is split and carefully elevated off of the middle phalanx base. The joint is now placed in flexion, and the extensor mechanism lateralizes allowing access to the joint surface (Fig. 12.7).

Proximal Phalanx Joint Surface and Intramedullary Canal Preparation

The joint surfaces are prepared for insertion of pyrolytic implant using the Ascension pyrolytic carbon PIP joint arthroplasty system (Austin, TX). The distal and proximal implant sizes used for this case were 10 and 20, respectively. A 0.035″ K-wire is inserted in the proximal phalanx head at the junction of the dorsal and middle third of the joint as viewed from a lateral perspective and centrally in a sagittal plane. This placement is confirmed with fluoroscopy and achieves a centralized starting point in the proximal phalanx. The K-wire is removed, and the hole enlarged using the Starter Awl to a size that will accommodate the Alignment Awl into the medul-

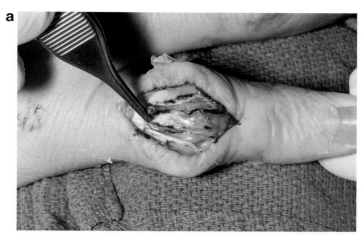

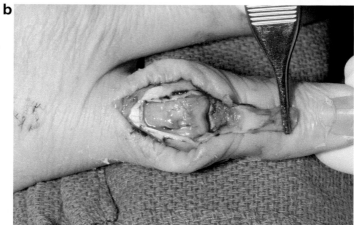

Fig. 12.6 (**a**) Chamay approach to the PIPJ with a distally based flap of extensor mechanism, preserving the insertion of the central slip. (**b**) Good visualization of the joint is possible with this approach

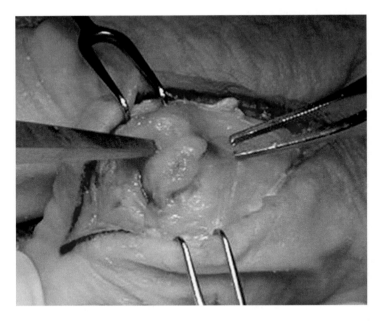

Fig. 12.7 Longitudinal extensor-splitting approach with lateral subluxation of extensor mechanism provides good access to the articular surface

lary canal. After placing the Alignment Awl, an Alignment Guide is attached. The Alignment Awl should be positioned parallel to the dorsal surface of the proximal phalanx and parallel with the long axis of the bone. Position should be fluoroscopically confirmed. The Alignment Guide is removed and replaced with the Vertical Cut Guide, which is positioned approximately 0.5–1.0 mm distal to the proximal attachments of the collateral ligaments. A micro-sagittal saw is used to remove the articular surface of the proximal phalanx, and the Alignment Awl removed. Offcuts can be saved for impaction grafting.

The proximal phalanx is then broached, with a goal of filling the intramedullary canal and maintaining a centralized alignment within the canal. This can be confirmed with fluoroscopic views. A burr is sometimes necessary to create an opening in very sclerotic bone, but

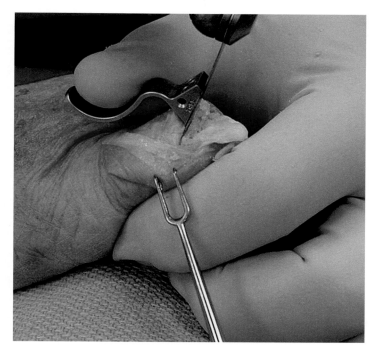

Fig. 12.8 Placement of the of oblique-cutting guide

burring should be minimized within the canal. Impaction grafting is recommended if burring is performed within the canal. In this case, a size 20 broach filled the medullary canal. Fluoroscopic imaging is important at this stage to ensure that the channel is centered within the intramedullary canal.

The last stage of joint surface preparation is to create an oblique volar cut of the proximal phalanx head. The Oblique Cut Guide the same size as the final broach is fully inserted into the medullary canal of the proximal phalanx. The guide must be seated against the vertical osteotomy. It is critical to ensure that there is no rotation of the Oblique Cut Guide, as this will ultimately lead to rotation of the final pyrolytic implant. A sagittal saw is placed flush with the guide to make the oblique cut (Fig. 12.8).

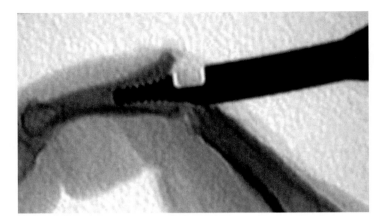

Fig. 12.9 Insertion of the distal broach in the middle phalanx filling the intramedullary canal

Middle Phalanx Joint Surface and Intramedullary Canal Preparation

With the joint hyperflexed, osteophytes are removed, and a 0.035″ K-wire is inserted into the junction of the dorsal and middle 1/3 of the base of the middle phalanx, confirming the position with X-ray. The distal component should not be placed too volar. The Starter Awl is next inserted, and the resultant hole further enlarged with a side-cutting burr until the defect is sufficient to accept the distal broach (Fig. 12.9). The articular surface is then removed with the side-cutting burr, preserving the central slip. A distal sizing template determines if the joint surface is smoothed sufficiently to allow for uniform seating of the implant. Like with the proximal component, the goal is to insert the largest implant possible with a centralized alignment. The distal component can be one size smaller or larger than the proximal component, but we would recommend matching the size of the proximal component.

Trial Insertion and Final Implant Selection

Appropriate-sized proximal and distal trials are placed. There should be full range of motion with stability upon lateral pressure and minimal laxity with traction. If there is laxity, a larger-sized proximal or distal component may be necessary. Prior to placing final implants, a fine K-wire should be used to create two dorsal holes on the middle phalanx base to allow for reattachment of the central slip as necessary. These sutures are placed before the final implant is placed. The final implants are then placed in the appropriate alignment. Final intraoperative radiographs are critical to ensure appropriate alignment.

Closure

The central slip is reconstructed with the sutures passed through the base of the middle phalanx to secure the flaps of extensor tendon to the distal insertion. The proximal extensor mechanism is repaired with 3.0 nonabsorbable sutures and the skin with nonabsorbable sutures. The dressing and splint should maintain slight PIP and DIP joint flexion and MP joint flexion of about 70° with both dorsal and volar support.

Technique Modifications for Hemiarthroplasty for Proximal Phalanx Resurfacing (Case 2)

The approach to the PIP joint is similar, but a small amount of central slip should be maintained at the base of the middle phalanx to allow for central slip reconstruction at the completion of the arthroplasty. Alternatively the central slip can be reattached through small bone tunnels in the middle phalanx. The central slip is repaired with a nonabsorbable, braided suture during closure. In the hemiarthroplasty case presented in this chapter, only the proximal phalanx was prepared, and this was done in the manner described above. A size 20 Ascension pyrolytic carbon implant (Austin, TX) was used.

References

1. Swanson AB, de Groot Swanson G. Flexible implant resection arthroplasty of the proximal interphalangeal joint. Hand Clin. 1994;10:261–6.
2. Brown AR, Claassen E. In situ analysis of antibody-forming cells from the BALB/c CRIc idiotype family: idiotopic heterogeneity among clustered cells. Cell Immunol. 1989;119:1–13.
3. Linscheid RL, Murray PM, Vidal MA, et al. Development of a surface replacement arthroplasty for proximal interphalangeal joints. J Hand Surg [Am]. 1997;22:286–98.
4. Beckenbaugh RD. Arthroplasty of the metacarpophalangeal joint using pyrocarbonate implants. Orthopade. 2003;32:794–7.
5. Cook SD, Beckenbaugh RD, Redondo J, et al. Long-term follow-up of pyrolytic carbon metacarpophalangeal implants. J Bone Joint Surg Am. 1999;81:635–48.
6. Integra. Integra PIPJ arthroplasty surgical technique guide. 14th edition. www.integralife.com.
7. Squitieri L, Chung KC. A systematic review of outcomes and complications of vascularized toe joint transfer, silicone arthroplasty, and PyroCarbon arthroplasty for posttraumatic joint reconstruction of the finger. Plast Reconstr Surg. 2008;121:1697–707.
8. Bravo CJ, Rizzo M, Hormel KB, et al. Pyrolytic carbon proximal interphalangeal joint arthroplasty: results with minimum two-year follow-up evaluation. J Hand Surg [Am]. 2007;32:1–11.
9. Nunley RM, Boyer MI, Goldfarb CA. Pyrolytic carbon arthroplasty for posttraumatic arthritis of the proximal interphalangeal joint. J Hand Surg [Am]. 2006;31:1468–74.

Chapter 13
PIP Fusion

Sidney M. Jacoby and Michael P. Gaspar

Abstract A healthy 42-year-old male presented to our clinic 10 weeks after sustaining an unstable PIP fracture-dislocation of his nondominant small finger. Radiographs revealed an impaction fracture along the volar base of P2 with persistent dorsal subluxation of the PIP joint. The patient's primary complaint was pain at the affected joint. He expressed a strong desire for treatment options that would minimize recovery time and need for future surgery, as his occupation as a tree surgeon required a quick return to work. The patient was treated with a primary arthrodesis of his left small finger PIP joint, as this offered a predictable and stable digit, pain relief, and a relatively quick return to work all while minimizing the potential for additional surgery in the future.

Keywords PIP • Fusion • Arthrodesis • Compression • Screw • Headless • Chronic • Fracture • Dislocation

S.M. Jacoby, M.D.
The Philadelphia Hand Center, P.C., Thomas Jefferson University
Department of Orthopaedic Surgery, 700 South Henderson
Road, Suite 200, King of Prussia, PA 19046, USA
e-mail: smjacoby@handcenters.com

M.P. Gaspar, M.D. (✉)
The Philadelphia Hand Center, P.C., Thomas Jefferson University
Department of Orthopaedic Surgery, The Franklin Building Suite G114,
834 Chestnut Street, Philadelphia, PA 19107, USA
e-mail: michaelpgaspar@gmail.com

© Springer International Publishing Switzerland 2016   171
J.E. Adams (ed.), *PIP Joint Fracture Dislocations*,
DOI 10.1007/978-3-319-28579-5_13

Case Presentation

A 42-year-old, right-hand dominant male presented to clinic 10 weeks after sustaining an injury to his left small finger. The patient described the event as a forced hyperextension against a large tree branch while working as a tree surgeon. Since the time of injury, he complained of persistent pain, swelling, and loss of motion at the PIP joint of the small finger. He also complained of subjective weakness of grip in the affected hand secondary to pain. He denied paresthesias and had only recently obtained health insurance which resulted in his delayed presentation. His past medical history and surgical history were unremarkable. He was self-employed as a tree surgeon and emphasized his desire to return to work as soon as possible. He denied any history of smoking or illicit drug use and drank alcohol on occasion.

Physical Assessment

Visual inspection of the patient's affected hand demonstrated obvious swelling and deformity at the PIP joint of the left small finger. The patient was unable to fully extend the PIP joint and had limited range of motion of the DIP joint. The PIP joint was tender to palpation, and passive range of motion at the joint elicited pain. Capillary refill and two-point discrimination at the fingertip were both within normal limits. Passive range of motion at the MCP and DIP joints were within normal range.

Diagnosis

Plain radiographs obtained of the left small finger revealed an impacted fracture along the volar base of the middle phalanx (P2) with persistent dorsal subluxation of the proximal phalanx (P1) (Fig. 13.1). The original fracture appeared to involve greater than 30 % of the base of the P2 joint surface.

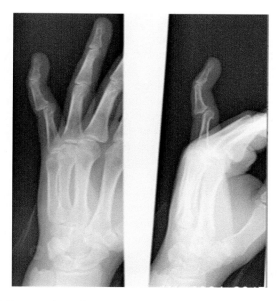

Fig. 13.1 Preoperative radiographs of left small finger demonstrate impacted fracture involving greater than 30 % of the volar lip of P2 with persistent dorsal subluxation of the PIP joint

Management Options

While a number of operative treatment options exist for an unstable fracture-dislocation at the PIP joint, the majority of these treatments, including open reduction and internal fixation (ORIF) with an interfragmentary screw, extension block splinting with pinning, and dynamic external fixation, have less utility in the face of a chronic injury, defined as greater than 6 weeks from the time of injury.

In the described scenario, and in general with chronic fractures and/or dislocations at the PIP joint, reasonable treatment options include hemi-hamate autograft arthroplasty (HHAA), total joint arthroplasty, volar plate arthroplasty (VPA), or arthrodesis. However, all arthroplasty options typically require an involved treatment and/or rehabilitation course to maintain adequate motion [2, 3, 17, 19]. In addition, the extent of soft-tissue and joint contraction that has already occurred due to delayed treatment may preclude the motion-sparing effects of these procedures. Furthermore, though hemi-hamate arthroplasty shows promising results with regard to short- and intermediate-term outcomes, it is a technically demanding procedure that can result in recurrent dislocation if the autograft is not properly oriented. While there are reports of success with delayed hemi-hamate arthroplasty, our patient was not interested in prolonged therapy with the possibility of future surgery [3, 8, 17, 19].

In the case of a chronic PIP injury, it is critically important to consider the patient's expectations and goals regarding the rehabilitation process and the long-term function of the finger involved. In this particular case, the patient was a motivated laborer, whose chief complaint was the pain associated with his injury. Furthermore, the injury involved his nondominant hand, and the patient was willing to forego motion if it allowed for faster return to work, minimal rehabilitation, and less potential need for follow-up visits or procedures. The decision was therefore to proceed with joint arthrodesis.

There are numerous surgical techniques designed to achieve a solid arthrodesis including: tension band constructs, K-wire fixation, compression screw fixation, and compression plating [4, 13, 18]. In considering the patient's desire for a quick postoperative recovery period, the authors felt that arthrodesis using a headless compression screw provided a good option while also limiting the drawbacks associated with the other techniques which may include pin tract problems, painful or prominent hardware, delayed union, and excessive soft-tissue dissection [6, 13, 14, 18].

Management Chosen

PIP joint fusion with headless compression screw.

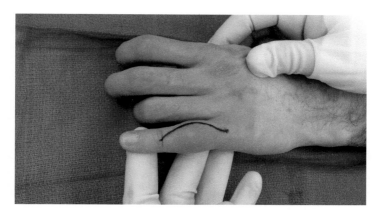

Fig. 13.2 Dorsal curvilinear incision for exposure over the PIP joint is *marked*

Clinical Course and Outcome

With the patient induced under general anesthesia, a pneumatic tourniquet was applied to the affected extremity. Preoperative antibiotics were utilized. A 3-cm dorsal curvilinear incision was made overlying the PIP joint (Fig. 13.2). Care was taken to preserve the dorsal venous supply. The combined structure of extensor tendon and PIP joint capsule was incised with particular attention to avoid detachment of the central slip from the base of the middle phalanx. Both collateral ligaments were released allowing for hyperflexion, or "shotgun" exposure of the PIP joint, maximizing bony exposure (Fig. 13.3). After osteophyte removal was performed using a rongeur, straight cuts using an oscillating saw were made according to the desired angle of fusion, which was planned preoperatively to correspond to a 30° position for optimal function. Close apposition of the bony surfaces was obtained prior to insertion of hardware. Once proper bony apposition was confirmed, an entry point for wire entry was marked roughly 1 cm from the joint line on the dorsal cortex of P1 using a surgical marking pen (Fig. 13.4). This is a critical step to protect the dorsal cortex from fragmentation

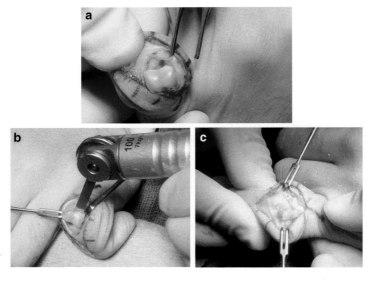

Fig. 13.3 (**a**) Collateral ligament release allows for hyperflexion or "shotgun" exposure of the PIP joint. (**b**) With the PIP joint in hyperflexion, the fusion surface is prepared using an oscillating saw. (**c**) After the cuts are made, adequate bony opposition is confirmed by direct inspection

during drilling. The wire was advanced into P2 at the desired angle of the arthrodesis in the sagittal plane, 30°. This was confirmed with lateral radiographs which revealed the wire to be in excellent orientation (Fig. 13.5). With the wire in place spanning the fusion site, a cannulated drill was then used over the guide wire to reach the cortical isthmus of the middle phalanx. After drilling, an opening reamer was used to enlarge the cortical hole on the dorsum of P1 to match the diameter of the trailing threads of the screw (Figs. 13.6 and 13.7). This critical step protects the dorsal cortex of P1 during screw insertion. The screw was then advanced until the leading end had engaged the isthmus of P2 and the proximal screw end was buried in the dorsal cortex of P1. This step is best optimized with an assistant holding the joint in firm compression, to ensure adequate compression and proper rotational alignment (Fig. 13.8).

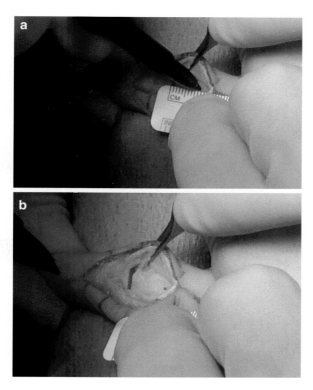

Fig. 13.4 (**a, b**) A ruler is used to measure and mark the insertion site for guide pin to be placed on the dorsal cortex of P1, approximately 1 cm proximal to the fusion site

Once proper alignment was confirmed with fluoroscopy, the extensor tendon was repaired with a 4-0 nonabsorbable suture using buried knots, and the skin was closed with 5-0 nylon sutures. A bulky dressing, with the hand splinted in the intrinsic plus position, was then applied (Figs. 13.9 and 13.10).

At 1-week follow-up, the patient had his surgical dressings and sutures removed and was transitioned to a PIP gutter splint (Fig. 13.11). The patient was instructed to keep the gutter splint on at all times (except for hand hygiene) until postoperative week 4. During

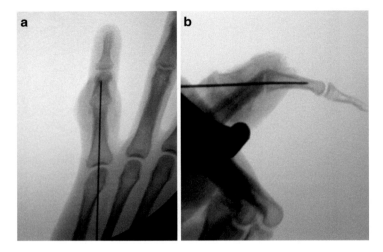

Fig. 13.5 (**a**) Anteroposterior and (**b**) lateral fluoroscopic images show pin placement perpendicular to fusion site while passing the isthmus of P2

that time, the patient was also encouraged to maintain range of motion for the other digits to prevent stiffness. The patient was cleared to resume resisted activities at 8 weeks when bony union was noted radiographically.

Clinical Pearls/Pitfalls

- Despite advances in both techniques and implants for small-joint arthroplasty of the digits, fusion remains a valuable treatment option for chronic fractures involving the PIP joint.
- Patients should be counseled about the potential trade-offs with regard to motion, function, stability, and complication rates when selecting fusion over arthroplasty.
- PIP fusion using headless compression screw provides a stable, pain-free construct with predictable union rates and minimal complications when performed correctly using meticulous attention to detail.

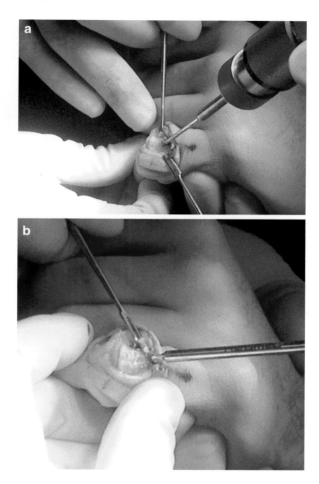

Fig. 13.6 (**a**) A drill is passed over the guide pin to the isthmus of P2. (**b**) An opening reamer is used to widen screw hole. Note the manual compression held by the assistant during drilling

- A curvilinear dorsal incision should be used for exposure; this minimizes potential for adhesions that may adversely affect extensor tendon function.
- Exposure of the joint is facilitated with incision of the combined extensor tendon and joint capsule structure at the

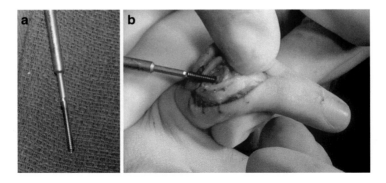

Fig. 13.7 (**a**) Headless compression screw prior to implantation. (**b**) Screw is placed across fusion site while assistant holds compression

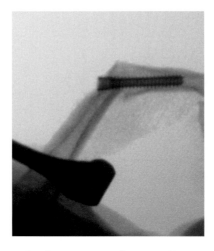

Fig. 13.8 Postoperative fluoroscopy confirms excellent screw placement on lateral view

level of the PIP with care taken to avoid detachment of the central slip from P2.
- Release of the collateral ligaments and excision of the volar plate allow for optimal hyperflexion or "shotgun" exposure to the joint surfaces.

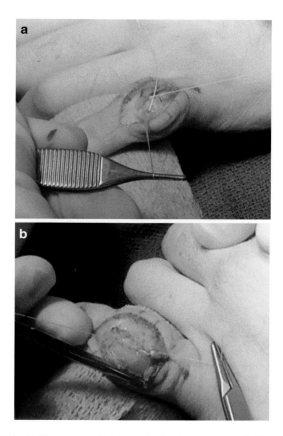

Fig. 13.9 (a, b) Extensor tendon is repaired using a nonabsorbable suture

- Once the fusion surfaces have been created with an oscillating saw, adequate opposition should be confirmed with manual inspection and manipulation of P1 and P2.
- It is critical for the insertion point of the guide pin to be roughly 1 cm proximal to the joint line to avoid disruption of the dorsal P1 cortex during drilling or screw placement.
- Drilling should be performed so as to at least reach the cortical isthmus of P2; this allows for screw fixation into the P2 isthmus for optimal fixation.

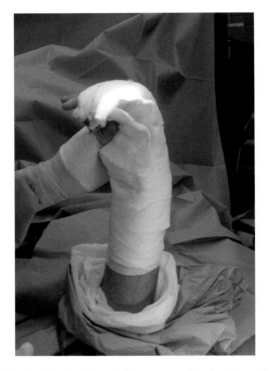

Fig. 13.10 Patient is placed in a bulky postoperative dressing with the hand splinted in the intrinsic plus position

- Prior to screw placement, the insertion hole in P1 should be enlarged to accommodate the trailing threads of the screw, again to protect the dorsal P1 cortex.
- Reduction should be held manually by an assistant, while screw is placed to ensure compression at the fusion site and proper rotational alignment.

Review of Literature and Discussion

Fracture-dislocations at the PIP joint of the finger involve a wide spectrum of characteristics that will typically dictate treatment options. In the case of acute injuries, the amount of joint surface

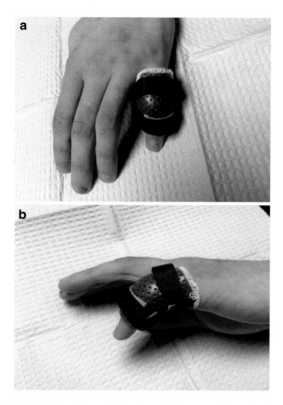

Fig. 13.11 (**a**, **b**) Patient is transitioned to a PIP gutter splint at the first follow-up visit, 1 week postoperatively

involved determines the stability of the joint and therefore dictates the need for surgical stabilization [7, 11]. If surgery is indicated, the intent is to restore functional motion and stability while improving pain patterns.

Chronic PIP fracture-dislocations present a more troublesome dilemma for the hand surgeon. In general, functional outcomes are far less predictable in treating chronic PIP injuries regardless of the technique chosen [7]. In addition, complication rates and need for additional surgeries tend to be higher for chronic cases [2, 9, 12]. Options are typically limited to arthroplasty or fusion, each with specific limitations and drawbacks.

Silicone implant arthroplasty has been described as a treatment option for chronic PIP fracture-dislocations, though data on its use in a population comprised exclusively of patients with chronic PIP fracture-dislocations is lacking [5]. Furthermore, there is a considerable failure rate of such implant arthroplasties even in the nontraumatic setting [11, 15]. When implant failure occurs, a salvage procedure via fusion is often the next option, but the potential for union may have been diminished by the index arthroplasty [10, 16]. The relatively newer, though technically challenging, hemi-hamate autograft arthroplasty technique shows promising results thus far. But again, like other methods for treatment of PIP fracture-dislocations, its outcomes when used in chronic injuries are worse than in acute injuries [3, 8]. It also has a variable rate of recurrent dislocation or subluxation, likely owing to its highly technical nature, which requires placement of a properly shaped, sized, and orientated autograft in order to restore the buttressing effect of the volar lip of P2.

The drawbacks of arthroplasty options induced the discussion of primary PIP arthrodesis as a treatment option for the chronic PIP fracture-dislocations presented in this case. With shared decision-making, we opted to proceed with primary fusion, thereby illustrating the important relationship between patient-dependant factors and selected treatment plan. Given the patient's occupation, an implant arthroplasty was likely to require future revision due to implant failure. In addition, because the injury was on the patient's nondominant hand, he was willing to compromise range of motion for pain relief. Perhaps most importantly, the patient desired the soonest possible return to work, with the least likelihood of need for further intervention in the future. As a result, with the predictably high union rate of arthrodesis and minimal concern for complications or need for revision procedures, joint fusion was a logical choice for our patient.

Following the decision to proceed with arthrodesis, our remaining task was to select from the number of available technique options. These options include K-wire fixation, tension band wiring, dorsal compression plating, and compression screw fixation. Though the use of K-wires or tension bands provide an effective yet relatively low-cost option, there are concerns regarding pin prominence and painful hardware, which in rare cases may require secondary surgery for hardware removal [1, 18]. In addition, there is a higher potential for delayed union requiring prolonged immobilization and/or activity restrictions [18]. Compression plating is not often the treatment of choice due to the extensive soft-tissue dissection required, with no distinct advantages over the other techniques [13].

Given the potential drawbacks of the other techniques, we preferred a headless compression screw which has shown excellent union rates in multiples studies, with superior clinical and biomechanical results when compared to other methods of PIP fusion [1, 4, 6, 13].

References

1. Breyer JM, Vergara P, Parra L, Sotelo P, Bifani A, Andrade F. Metacarpophalangeal and interphalangeal joint arthrodesis: a comparative study between tension band and compression screw fixation. J Hand Surg Eur Vol. 2015;40:374. doi:10.1177/1753193413514362.
2. Burton RI, Campolattaro RM, Ronchetti PJ. Volar plate arthroplasty for osteoarthritis of the proximal interphalangeal joint: a preliminary report. J Hand Surg Am. 2002;27:1065–72. doi:10.1053/jhsu.2002.35871.
3. Calfee RP, Kiefhaber TR, Sommerkamp TG, Stern PJ. Hemi-hamate arthroplasty provides functional reconstruction of acute and chronic proximal interphalangeal fracture-dislocations. J Hand Surg Am. 2009;34(7):1232–41. doi:10.1016/j.jhsa.2009.04.027.
4. Capo JT, Melamed E, Shamian B, et al. Biomechanical evaluation of 5 fixation devices for proximal interphalangeal joint arthrodesis. J Hand Surg Am. 2014;39(10):1971–7. doi:10.1016/j.jhsa.2014.07.035.
5. Criner KT, Ilyas AM. Silicone arthroplasty for chronic proximal interphalangeal joint dislocations. Tech Hand Up Extrem Surg. 2011;15(4):209–14. doi:10.1097/BTH.0b013e31820f8b53.
6. Deitch MA, Kiefhaber TR, Comisar BR, Stern PJ. Original communications: dorsal fracture dislocations of the proximal interphalangeal joint: surgical complications and long-term results. J Hand Surg Am. 1999;24(A):914–23.
7. Elfar J, Mann T. Fracture-dislocations of the proximal interphalangeal joint. J Am Acad Orthop Surg. 2013;21:88–98. doi:10.5435/JAAOS-21-02-88.
8. Frueh FS, Calcagni M, Lindenblatt N. The hemi-hamate autograft arthroplasty in proximal interphalangeal joint reconstruction: a systematic review. J Hand Surg Eur Vol. 2014;40:24–32. doi:10.1177/1753193414554356.

9. Grant I, Berger AC, Tham SKY. Internal fixation of unstable fracture dislocations of the proximal interphalangeal joint. J Hand Surg Am.
   2005;30(5):492–8. doi:10.1016/j.jhsb.2005.05.006.

10. Jones DB, Ackerman DB, Sammer DM, Rizzo M. Arthrodesis as a salvage
    for failed proximal interphalangeal joint arthroplasty. J Hand Surg Am.
    2011;36(2):259–64. doi:10.1016/j.jhsa.2010.10.030.

11. Kang R, Stern PJ. Fracture dislocations of the proximal interphalangeal
    joint. J Am Soc Surg Hand. 2002;2(2):47–59. doi:10.1053/jssh.2002.33317.

12. Kiefhaber TR, Stern PI. Clinical perspective fracture dislocations of the
    proximal interphalangeal joint. J Hand Surg Am. 1998;23A:368–80.

13. Leibovic SJ, Strickland JW. Arthrodesis of the proximal interphalangeal
    joint of the finger: comparison of the use of the Herbert screw with other
    fixation methods. J Hand Surg Am. 1994;19:181–8. doi:10.1016/0363-
    5023(94)90002-7.

14. Leibovic SJ. Arthrodesis of the interphalangeal joints with headless
    compression screws. J Hand Surg Am. 2007;32:1113–9. doi:10.1016/j.
    jhsa.2007.06.010.

15. Mikolyzk DK, Stern PJ. Steinmann pin arthrodesis for salvage of failed
    small joint arthroplasty. J Hand Surg Am. 2011;36(8):1383–7. doi:10.1016/j.
    jhsa.2011.05.027.

16. Pritsch T, Rizzo M. Reoperations following proximal interphalangeal joint
    nonconstrained arthroplasties. J Hand Surg Am. 2011;36(9):1460–6.
    doi:10.1016/j.jhsa.2011.06.002.

17. Tyser AR, Tsai MA, Parks BG, Means KR. Biomechanical characteristics
    of hemi-hamate reconstruction versus volar plate arthroplasty in the treat-
    ment of dorsal fracture dislocations of the proximal interphalangeal joint.
    J Hand Surg Am. 2015;40(2):329–32. doi:10.1016/j.jhsa.2014.10.061.

18. Uhl RL. Proximal interphalangeal joint arthrodesis using the tension
    band technique. J Hand Surg Am. 2007;32(3):914–7. doi:10.1016/j.
    jhsa.2007.04.014.

19. Williams RMM, Kiefhaber TR, Sommerkamp TG, Stern PJ. Treatment of
    unstable dorsal proximal interphalangeal fracture/dislocations using a
    hemi-hamate autograft. J Hand Surg Am. 2003;28(03):856–65. doi:10.1016/
    S0363-5023(03)00304-6.

Suggested Readings

Leibovic SJ. Arthrodesis of the interphalangeal joints with headless compression screws. J Hand Surg Am. 2007;32:1113–9. doi:10.1016/j.
   jhsa.2007.06.010.

Leibovic SJ, Strickland JW. Arthrodesis of the proximal interphalangeal joint
   of the finger: comparison of the use of the Herbert screw with other
   fixation methods. J Hand Surg Am. 1994;19:181–8.
   doi:10.1016/0363-5023(94)90002-7.

Chapter 14
Pediatric PIP Joint Injuries

Felicity G. Fishman

Abstract Pediatric proximal interphalangeal joint dislocations occur infrequently in comparison to pediatric finger fractures secondary to the anatomy of the skeletally immature hand. Although majority of pediatric PIP joint dislocations can be successfully treated with closed reduction, more complex or unstable injuries (crush injuries, fracture-dislocations) may require open reduction and fixation for improved stability. Closed treatment in children may warrant sedation in addition to a local anesthetic. Outcomes following reduction are generally favorable with stiffness occurring more commonly following a volar PIP dislocation than a dorsal dislocation. Complications include persistent instability, stiffness, and premature physeal closure.

Keywords Proximal interphalangeal joint • Pediatric • Physis • Premature physeal arrest

Abbreviations

PIP   Proximal interphalangeal
MCP   Metacarpophalangeal

F.G. Fishman, M.D. (✉)
Yale Orthopaedics & Rehabilitation,
PO Box 208701, New Haven, CT 06520, USA
e-mail: felicity.fishman@yale.edu

© Springer International Publishing Switzerland 2016   187
J.E. Adams (ed.), *PIP Joint Fracture Dislocations*,
DOI 10.1007/978-3-319-28579-5_14

Pathoanatomy

Hand injuries in children are quite common, accounting for a significant number of annual visits to the pediatric emergency department [1]. The hand is one of the most frequently injured portions of the body in children, particularly vulnerable as children explore the world around them with their fingers [2]. In the skeletally immature hand, the strength of the soft tissue structures (collateral ligaments, volar plate, tendons) exceeds the strength of the adjacent physis. Therefore, physeal and epiphyseal injuries tend to occur more commonly than failure of the tendons and/or ligaments [3, 4]. In the proximal interphalangeal joint (PIP), the collateral ligaments originate from the collateral recess of the proximal phalangeal head and insert on the metaphysis and epiphysis of the middle phalanx and the volar plate, spanning the physis. This portends stability of the epiphysis and physis against laterally directed forces but often results in fractures of the metaphysis, consistent with a Salter Harris II injury pattern [3, 4]. Despite the relative strength discrepancy between the soft tissue structures and the physis, dislocations and fracture-dislocations of the interphalangeal joints do occur.

Presentation

PIP dislocations are relatively uncommon in younger children but are seen more frequently in the adolescent athlete population [5]. Depending on the age of the injured child, physical examination may be complicated by a lack of communication, by inability to follow commands, and by fear and anxiety. After a thorough physical examination, radiographic evaluation of the injured digit should be performed. Radiographs in children can be challenging to interpret secondary to ossification patterns and lack of fine bony detail visible on the imaging [4]. In very young children, fractures associated with dislocations can be missed secondary to lack of ossification of the epiphysis. It is imperative to obtain a true lateral of the affected finger, and not the hand, to properly evaluate the congruency of the PIP joint. This is particularly important following reduction of the dislocation in order to evaluate for residual subluxation of the PIP joint, which can result in a radiolucent "V" dorsally in lieu of a symmetric arc [6].

Pathology

Pediatric PIP dislocations can occur dorsally, volarly, and laterally. Mechanisms of injury include axial load with hyperextension, flexion, or rotation of the PIP joint. Alternatively, PIP dislocations can occur secondary to crush injuries, particularly in younger children [7]. Similar to the incidence in adults, dorsal dislocations are the most common. Dorsal dislocations generally occur due to a hyperextension force with disruption of the collateral ligaments and volar plate, resulting in the middle phalanx displaced dorsally to the proximal phalanx.

Volar dislocations are less common than dorsal dislocations and can be more difficult to reduce. The mechanism of injury is generally an axial force with a rotational component acting upon the partially flexed middle phalanx. The middle phalanx rests volar to the proximal phalanx with an injury sustained to the collateral ligaments, central slip insertion, and often an accompanying fracture. The entire epiphysis or fractured portion of the epiphysis may block reduction of the PIP joint [8]. Lateral PIP dislocations occur far less commonly than dorsal dislocations, although dorsal dislocations may have a lateral component. A pure lateral dislocation is a secondary to disruption of the proper and accessory collateral ligaments as well as the volar plate. Radiographs may demonstrate bony avulsion fractures, indicative of ligamentous and volar plate disruptions [4].

Treatment

Treatment of pediatric PIP dislocations initially consists of attempted closed reduction. Many dorsal dislocations may be partial collateral/volar plate injuries with subluxation of the middle phalanx, which are reduced prior to arrival in the emergency department. Closed reduction can be aided by the administration of analgesia in older children and analgesia supplemented by sedation in younger children. A teenager may tolerate administration of a digital anesthetic without sedation, but younger children may require intranasal or intravenous sedation for proper control of pain and anxiety prior to administration of a local block or reduction maneuvers [9, 10].

After the child is properly anesthetized, likely with a digital block supplemented by sedation, the metacarpophalangeal (MCP) joints and wrist should be flexed to take tension off the flexor tendons. The reduction maneuver then consists of gentle longitudinal traction, followed by translation of the middle phalanx (volarly for a dorsal dislocation and dorsally for a volar dislocation) onto the proximal phalanx [4, 8]. A mini C-arm can be utilized to help assess the congruity of the joint and stability of the reduction. The PIP joint should be taken through a range of motion following reduction to confirm stability, with particular attention paid to any subtle dorsal subluxation in extension after reduction of a dorsal dislocation. If the PIP joint remains unstable in 30° or more of flexion, operative stabilization (K-wire, external fixation) should be considered [11].

If the dislocation is irreducible, open reduction should be performed. Volar dislocations are more commonly irreducible than dorsal dislocations. This may be secondary to interposition of the phalangeal head within the soft tissues, interposition of the soft tissues within the joint or bony fragments of the epiphysis that block reduction (Fig. 14.1a–c). Multiple attempts at closed reduction should not be performed in a child secondary to the risk of increased trauma to the physis. The operative approach to the digit can be dorsal, volar, or mid-axial, depending on the preference of the surgeon and the direction of the displacement and/or incarcerated fragments. Irreducible volar dislocations are typically approached dorsally with repair of the central slip following reduction. Kirschner wire fixation may be used to temporarily immobilize the PIP and secure fracture fixation following reduction.

Following closed reduction of a simple dorsal dislocation, the finger should be briefly splinted for comfort (3–7 days) and then gentle range of motion initiated. Buddy taping or straps can be utilized to

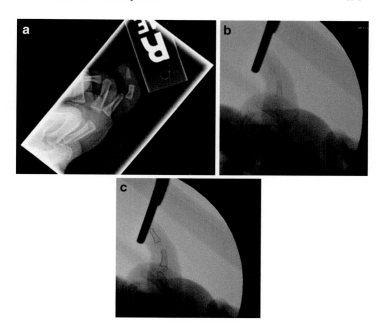

Fig. 14.1 (**a**) Crush injury to the hand of a 9-month-old child with PIP and DIP dislocations. (**b**) Fluoroscopic image after attempted closed reduction. PIP joint is irreducible due to transphyseal fracture. (**c**) Drawing schematic demonstrating transphyseal fracture with displaced unossified epiphysis. Patient underwent open reduction of dislocation and pinning of digit

help protect the collateral ligaments and volar plate during early motion and to provide the child with a sense of stability as they begin to mobilize the digit. If instability is noted within 30° (or less) of full extension following reduction of a dorsal dislocation, an extension block splint should be fashioned. The AlumaFoam splint is placed as an outrigger from a short arm cast to ensure compliance with splinting in the pediatric population.

If a volar dislocation is successfully reduced in a closed fashion, the PIP joint should be protected for 4 weeks in full extension to allow healing of the injured central slip. In an older child, this may be accomplished with an AlumaFoam or therapist-fashioned orthoplast splint. In younger children, an AlumaFoam splint should be supplemented with a cast. Lateral dislocations are typically successfully reduced in a closed fashion and can be protected with 5–7 days of immobilization followed by early motion with buddy straps or buddy taping.

Outcomes/Complications

Simple dorsal dislocations that are successfully reduced in a closed fashion generally have favorable outcomes with an early motion protocol. Volar dislocations and more complex or unstable dorsal fracture-dislocations have less favorable prognoses. Missed injuries that present late with subluxation of the middle phalanx often result in considerable stiffness of the PIP joint and may require delayed capsular release to improve motion. Complications also include premature physeal arrest of the middle phalanx particularly in PIP fracture-dislocations.

Case Example

An 11-year-old right-hand-dominant male presented to the pediatric emergency room for evaluation of his left hand following an injury that occurred while playing basketball. He had swelling and an obvious deformity of his left small finger. Radiographs demonstrated a dorsolateral dislocation of his left small finger PIP joint without an obvious fracture (Fig. 14.2a, b). The child was placed supine on the hospital stretcher with his left arm abducted to his side. He was provided with oral analgesia prior to administration of a digital block (1 % lidocaine without epinephrine). A careful sensory exam was performed prior to the digital block. With the wrist and MCP joints flexed, gentle longitudinal traction was applied to the small finger, and the middle phalanx was translated volarly and radially to reduce the PIP joint. Fluoroscopic images were obtained at the bedside to confirm congruent reduction and stability throughout a full range of motion. Formal post-reduction radiographs were obtained to confirm a symmetric PIP joint reduction

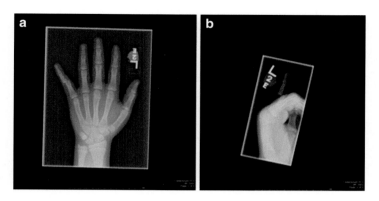

Fig. 14.2 (**a**, **b**) PA and lateral view of an 11-year-old boy with left small finger PIP dislocation

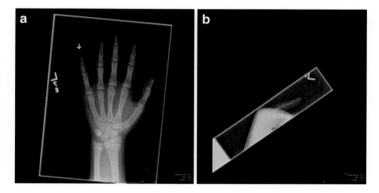

Fig. 14.3 (**a**, **b**) Small finger of an 11-year-old boy status post-closed reduction of left small finger dorsolateral PIP dislocation

(Fig. 14.3a, b). The patient was placed in a short arm ulnar gutter plaster splint in the intrinsic plus position. Five days following his injury, he was evaluated in the clinic and transitioned from the cast to buddy straps between the ring and small fingers. At 6 weeks following injury, he had full small finger PIP extension and could make a composite fist despite mild residual swelling about the PIP joint. He was able to return to basketball at this time without discomfort with continued buddy taping.

Conclusion

Pediatric PIP joint dislocations are relatively uncommon secondary to the strength of the volar plate and collateral ligaments in comparison to the physis in the skeletally immature hand. Dorsal dislocations occur most frequently and typically can be reduced in a closed fashion followed by a short period of splinting and early mobilization. Unstable dorsal dislocations are best treated with extension block splinting or pinning. Volar dislocations are often more challenging to reduce and can have less favorable outcomes plagued by stiffness and premature physeal arrest. Special consideration should be given to sedation prior to administration of digital anesthetics in younger children as well as to casting for postreduction immobilization to improve compliance in the pediatric population.

References

1. Bhende M, Dandrea L, Davis H. Hand injuries in children presenting to a pediatric emergency department. Ann Emerg Med. 1993;20(10):1519–23.
2. Hastings H, Simmons B. Hand fractures in children. A statistical analysis. Clin Orthop Relat Res. 1984;188:120–30.
3. Hankin F, Janda H. Tendon and ligament attachments in relationship to growth plates in a child's hand. J Hand Surg Br. 1989;14-B:315–8.
4. Kozin SH, Waters PM. Fractures and dislocations of the hand and carpus in children. In: Beaty JH, Kasser JR, editors. Rockwood and Wilkins' fractures in children. 6th ed. Philadelphia, PA: Lippincott Williams & Wilkins; 2006. p. 257–336.
5. Flynn JM, Skaggs DL, Waters PM. Staying out of trouble while treating hand, wrist, and forearm injury. In: Skaggs DL, Flynn JM, editors. Staying out of trouble in pediatric orthopaedics. Philadelphia, PA: Lippincott Williams & Wilkins; 2006. p. 80–95.
6. Calfee RP, Sommerkamp TG. Fracture-dislocation about the finger joints. J Hand Surg Am. 2009;34A:1140–7.
7. Wenger DR, Pring ME. Hand. In: Rang M, Pring ME, Wenget DR, editors. Rang's children's fractures. 3rd ed. Philadelphia, PA: Lippincott Williams & Wilkins; 2005. p. 151–65.

8. Jones N, Jupiter J. Irreducible palmar dislocation of the proximal interphalangeal joint associated with an epiphyseal fracture in the middle phalanx. J Hand Surg Am. 1985;10A(2):261–4.
9. McCarty EC, Mencio GA, Green NE. Anesthesia and analgesia for the ambulatory management of fractures in children. J Am Acad Orthop Surg. 1999;7:81–91.
10. Pizzo JD, Callahan J. Intranasal medications in pediatric emergency medicine. Pediatr Emerg Care. 2014;30:496–504.
11. Kiefhaber TR, Stern PJ. Fracture dislocations of the proximal interphalangeal joint. J Hand Surg Am. 1998;23A(3):368–80.

Chapter 15
Nonoperative Treatment of Volar PIP Joint Fracture Dislocations

Alex J. Ferikes, Scott W. Rogers, C. Liam Dwyer, John D. Lubahn, Terri L. Wolfe, and Katie Froehlich

Abstract Volar proximal interphalangeal (PIP) joint fracture-dislocations are not commonly described in the literature; even more infrequently discussed is the nonoperative management of these injuries. The mechanism of injury typically involves an axial load with associated hyperextension of the PIP joint (Kiefhaber and Stern. J Hand Surg Am. 23:368–380, 1998). These injuries can also be referred to as dorsal lip injuries (Kang and Stern. J Am Acad Orthop Surg. 2:47–59, 2002) referring to the anatomic site of insertion to the central slip of the dorsal apparatus of the extensor mechanism in the "dorsal lip" of the articular surface of the middle phalanx at the PIPJ. The classification system typically used for these injuries is stable versus unstable, referring to the examination of the PIPJ following reduction of the articular surface with

A.J. Ferikes, M.D. • S.W. Rogers, M.D. • C.L. Dwyer, M.D.
J.D. Lubahn, M.D.
Department of Orthopaedic Surgery, UPMC Hamot,
201 State Street, Erie, PA 16550, USA

T.L. Wolfe, O.T.R./L., C.H.T. (✉) • K. Froehlich, O.T.R./L., C.H.T.
Hand and Upper Body Rehabilitation Center,
300 State Street, Erie, PA 16507, USA
e-mail: TerriWolfe@eriehandcenter.com

© Springer International Publishing Switzerland 2016
J.E. Adams (ed.), *PIP Joint Fracture Dislocations*,
DOI 10.1007/978-3-319-28579-5_15

the joint held in full extension (Kiefhaber and Stern. J Hand Surg Am. 23:368–380, 1998). These injuries, while infrequent, may present similarly to other PIP joint injuries, in a delayed fashion, as a "jammed" or "sprained" finger (Kiefhaber and Stern. J Hand Surg Am. 23:368–380, 1998). Early recognition and treatment of these injuries can improve outcomes. Regardless of whether operative or nonoperative treatment is pursued, the main principles of treatment include obtaining and maintaining a concentric joint reduction and restoration of joint stability and implementation of early motion (Kang and Stern. J Am Acad Orthop Surg. 2:47–59, 2002). Nonoperative management is typically only considered for stable injuries with less than 2 mm of fracture displacement with the mainstay of treatment in these cases being static immobilization (Kiefhaber and Stern. J Hand Surg Am. 23:368–380, 1998). These patients require close monitoring and frequent radiographic follow-up to ensure maintenance of reduction (Kiefhaber and Stern. J Hand Surg Am. 23:368–380, 1998). Our case presentation presented in this chapter highlights the clinician's ability to achieve a satisfactory outcome using nonoperative management in volar PIP joint fracture-dislocations.

Keywords Volar proximal interphalangeal joint fracture-dislocation • Volar PIP joint fracture-dislocation • Nonoperative management of volar PIP joint fracture-dislocation

Typical Mechanism of Injury

The PIP joint is vulnerable to injury due to its long moment arm and relatively unprotected position. Middle phalangeal fractures are typically caused by avulsion or impaction-shear mechanisms; however, these volar PIP joint fracture-dislocations often result from an axial load with a hyperextension element at the joint as well [1, 2]. Another described mechanism of injury involves an axial load with an associated palmarly directed force on the middle phalanx base [3]. Other authors have described the mechanism of injury as occurring from a rotatory longitudinal force on a semiflexed digit [4, 5]. Forced PIP joint hyperflexion may lead to central tendon disruption that can be intrasubstance or an avulsion from the middle phalanx [2].

Clinical Evaluation and Imaging

Clinical evaluation begins with a thorough, yet focused, history and physical examination. One key historical element to ascertain is the time from injury to presentation, as many of these patients may not seek treatment initially. The delay may be due to bystanders treating presumed simple "dislocations," and in these cases there is no initial radiographic evaluation [4, 6].

The physical examination should include inspection of the skin and notation of obvious deformities, open injuries, bruising, edema, malrotation, or malalignment [6]. Any skin puckering may be indicative of interposed soft-tissue structures [7]. The evaluation of joint range of motion (ROM) and stability is essential, but may require the use of a digital nerve block depending on patient comfort. Once properly anesthetized, if needed, both active and passive ROM can be evaluated. At this point the collateral ligaments should be tested, giving further indication of joint stability [4, 8]. If subluxation occurs with active motion, there should be a high suspicion for either major ligament disruption or a large intra-articular joint fracture [4]. Translation of the middle phalanx dorsally indicates a torn volar plate [6]. An Elson test should be used to assess central slip integrity. In this maneuver the digit is flexed at the PIP joint, and the patient is asked to extend the distal interphalangeal (DIP) joint against resistance. If the DIP joint can actively extend, the integrity of the central slip is compromised. If the DIP joint remains "floppy" and cannot fully extend, the central slip is intact [9].

Initial imaging should include standard AP and lateral X-rays centered on the PIP joint of the affected digit. Traction X-rays or a CT scan may be particularly helpful to more completely evaluate the presence and extent of a depressed articular fracture [6].

After images of the injured digit have been obtained, a reduction maneuver should be attempted if the joint is subluxed or dislocated. Longitudinal traction and a dorsally directed force on the base of the middle phalanx are usually sufficient to reduce the joint. Stress X-rays are not typically needed for diagnosis of collateral instability; however, they may be useful to document the extent of instability. While performing a varus and valgus stress on the joint, it is important to note the end points of the ligaments [4].

There are times when volar fracture-dislocations are irreducible. The most common cause of irreducibility is when the proximal phalanx becomes entrapped in the dorsal extensor apparatus [12]. Alternatively the lateral bands or the collateral ligaments with or without an attached bony fragment may become interposed in the joint [10–12]. Prior to reduction a careful physical exam may help identify skin puckering, which is a good indication that there is soft tissue interposed in the joint [7]. These instances warrant an open reduction in a timely manner [6].

Classification

Most commonly, volar PIP joint fracture-dislocations are classified as stable vs. unstable [1, 2, 4, 6]. Stable fractures are described as those that exhibit no palmar subluxation when the PIP joint is placed into full extension. The fracture of the base of the middle phalanx typically involves less than 50 % of the joint surface. A lateral X-ray with the digit in full extension is used to confirm joint reduction. Unstable fracture-dislocations are those with any degree palmar translation of the middle phalanx when the PIP joint is in extension, regardless of the size of the fracture or degree of comminution [1].

A less commonly cited classification system may be used for dorsal lip fractures. These are classified from I to III [4]. Type I involves <25 % of the articular surface with no associated subluxation of the middle phalanx. Type II involves <50 % of the articular surface with or without mild subluxation of the middle phalanx. Type III occurs with any size dorsal lip fracture with complete palmar dislocation of the middle phalanx [4].

Treatment Options

Initial management of these injuries often occurs outside of a healthcare setting, such as on a field of play, often by the patient or another bystander [13]. If the patient presents while still dislocated, a digital block with local anesthesia may be helpful to reduce the fracture, followed by axial traction and a dorsally directed force over the middle phalanx. Sometimes, however, the closed reduction may not be achieved easily. A "milking" type maneuver, working from proximal to distal, may aid reduction by decreasing tension on the extrinsic flexor and extensor tendons at the joint. Avoid multiple attempts at closed reduction if it is grossly unstable or difficult to reduce [14]. Indications for an open reduction include the following: inability to achieve concentric reduction, soft-tissue interposition, or displacement of dorsal lip fracture >1 mm from its anatomic position.

There are numerous treatment options for these injuries. Nonoperative management typically consists of static immobilization. There has not been much change in the treatment of these injuries recently according to Shah et al. [3]. The largest series reported is by Rosenstadt et al. [10], which consisted of 13 patients, nine acute and four chronic. Treatment included closed reduction with percutaneous pin fixation, open reduction internal fixation, and open reduction and soft-tissue reconstruction. Other operative options include longitudinal traction devices or static immobilization using a K-wire [1, 15].

Treatment Considerations

Indications for operative treatment are essentially in line with the simple classification scheme of stable versus unstable injuries. Stable fracture patterns, those that remain reduced in full extension, may be good candidates for nonoperative treatment with static immobilization. The main goal is to reestablish central tendon continuity. Up to a 2 mm displacement of the dorsal central slip avulsion fracture can still yield good results [1, 2].

Unstable fracture patterns will generally require operative management. Any subluxation of the joint with full extension is an indication for operative management in order to restore joint congruity and a concentric reduction. Another reason why nonoperative management is not considered for unstable fracture-dislocations is that they would require a prolonged period of immobilization, and significant permanent stiffness can occur [13]. Patient compliance with either postoperative rehabilitation or nonoperative treatment should also be factored when choosing a treatment pathway.

Nonoperative Treatment Protocol/Algorithm

Only stable PIP joint fracture-dislocations, as described above, should be considered for nonoperative treatment. Exceptions to this include patients who are unwilling or unable to undergo surgical fixation.

The PIP joint is immobilized in full extension for 3–4 weeks [1, 16]. The main goal of immobilization is to regain and maintain central slip tendon continuity [1]. When the central slip is disrupted, the FDS pull is unopposed on the base of the middle phalanx in a volar direction, leading to possible subluxation or dislocation [2]. The PIP joint only is to be immobilized while the DIP joint is left free for active and passive ROM [1]. At 4 weeks the patient is then placed into dynamic extension splinting that allows for active flexion. At 6 weeks passive flexion and strengthening are begun. However, splinting should continue for 6–8 weeks total, with the patient placed back into immobilization when not engaged in therapy [16]. With PIP joint flexion, maintenance of reduction can be lost due to reduced strength of the extensors compared to the flexors or due to sub-tendinous adhesions causing inadequate extensor excursion proximally [4]. Serial imaging should be obtained to monitor maintenance of reduction, beginning with weekly X-rays for the first 2–3 weeks.

Return to full activity should be delayed until the patient has no tenderness to palpation at the fracture site, and X-rays show consolidation at the fracture. Ideally, the patient should also be at their

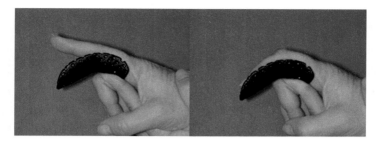

Fig. 15.1 Template to gradually gain flexion while preserving active extension

maximal post-treatment range of motion. Regarding sport specific return to play, Birman and Rossenwasser recommend baseball players return to batting when full and painless grip are possible and that pitchers must wait until completely healed before beginning a throwing program. Skeletally immature players are protected until healing is confirmed clinically and radiographically [14].

Indications for Therapy

Referral to therapy is indicated when there are limitations in active and passive range of motion. If the central slip is intact, the PIPJ has been immobilized in extension. As AROM is allowed, there typically is a lack of flexion at the PIP joint. Motion toward flexion is the goal but not at risk of losing PIPJ extension. If the joint is unstable, a static orthosis or cast is prescribed. An exercise template helps to educate the patient on the degree of flexion allowed without causing instability (Fig. 15.1).

If there is a closed reduction, but the central slip is ruptured, the typical immobilization is between 4 and 6 weeks with serial cast or finger gutter orthosis (Fig. 15.2), supporting as much extension as possible. The orthosis is removed for hygiene only and the joint evaluated for the development of an extension lag. At 4–6 weeks a controlled motion program is initiated, and a hand-based or finger-based dynamic PIP extension orthotic is recommended (Fig. 15.3).

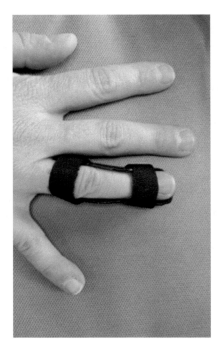

Fig. 15.2 Gutter orthosis

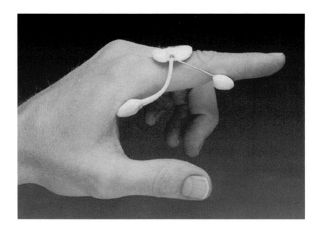

Fig. 15.3 Dynamic DeRoyal® LMB PIP joint extension orthosis

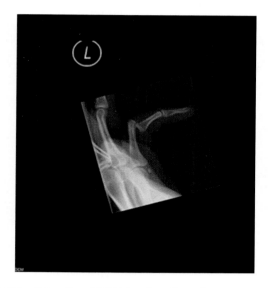

Fig. 15.4 Volar dislocation of PIP joint via radiograph

Use of a finger extension orthotic at night maintains the gains made during the day. Typically AROM of the PIP joint is started at 4 weeks if there is no extension lag and may begin even earlier.

Case Study

A 17-year-old female was injured playing soccer. She sustained a left small finger PIP joint volar dislocation during a soccer game as verified on radiograph (Fig. 15.4). She was seen in a rural ER where her PIPJ was reduced and splinted in full extension. During the subsequent weeks of her treatment, she began to develop a pseudo-boutonniere deformity (Fig. 15.5). She attended therapy 2–3 times per week for 6 weeks before being referred to a hand surgery practice and subsequently to a certified hand therapist

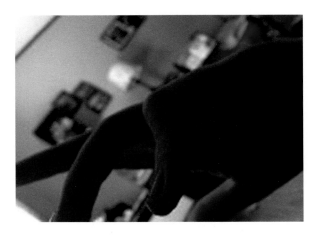

Fig. 15.5 Volar dislocation of PIPJ

(CHT). Her clinical exam revealed a stiff PIP joint with pain when mobilized into full extension. A hard end feel was noted and her active motion was as follows (in degrees): MP 0–90, PIP 60–85, and DIP +15–25. She underwent 7 weeks of therapy including serial casting, joint mobilization, oblique retinacular ligament (ORL) stretching, joint blocking, and reverse blocking exercises (Figs. 15.6, 15.7, 15.8, 15.9, and 15.10). Gains were made in PIP extension. At the end of her therapy course, active motion was as follows: MP 0–90, PIP 25–70, and DIP 0–40 (Fig. 15.11).

Summary

Volar fracture-dislocations of the PIP joint are uncommon injuries; however, there are indications for nonoperative management. If the injuries are considered stable after reduction, they are likely amenable to nonoperative treatment. The mainstays of nonoperative management are static immobilization initially in order to maintain a concentric reduction of the joint and close follow-up.

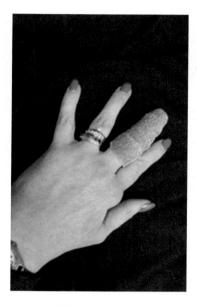

Fig. 15.6 Serial casting into PIP extension

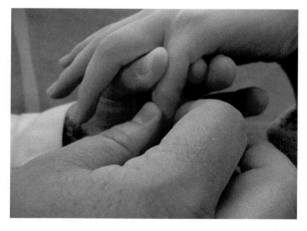

Fig. 15.7 PIPJ mobilization to regain extension

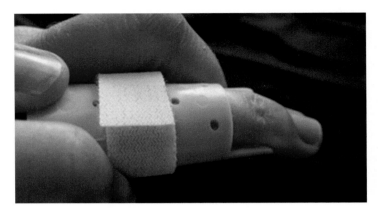

Fig. 15.8 Isolating the DIP to lengthen the ORL

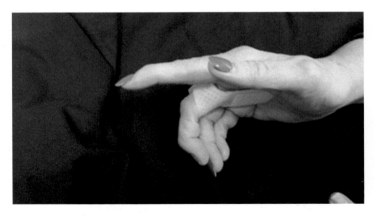

Fig. 15.9 Use of an orthosis to isolate the PIPJ. This "blocking" exercise can also be done manually

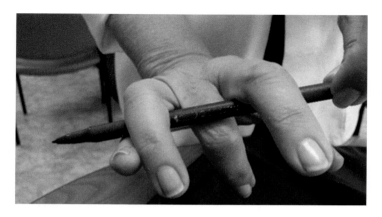

Fig. 15.10 "Reverse blocking" via use of a pen. This may also be done manually or through the use of a relative motion (RM) orthosis

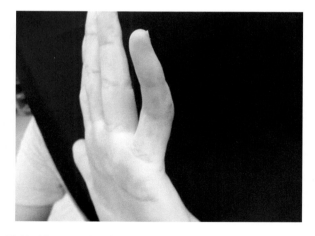

Fig. 15.11 After 7 weeks of treatment by a CHT

References

1. Kiefhaber TR, Stern PJ. Fracture dislocations of the proximal interphalangeal joint. J Hand Surg Am. 1998;23:368–80. doi:10.1016/S0363-5023(05)80454-X.

2. Kang R, Stern PJ. Fracture dislocations of the proximal interphalangeal joint. J Am Acad Orthop Surg. 2002;2:47–59. doi:10.1053/jssh.2002.33317.

3. Shah CM, Sommerkamp TG. Fracture dislocation of the finger joints. J Hand Surg Am. 2014;39:792–802. doi:10.1016/j.jhsa.2013.10.001.

4. Chinchalkar SJ, Gan BS. Management of proximal interphalangeal joint fractures and dislocations. J Hand Ther. 2003;16:117–28. doi:10.1016/S0894-1130(03)80007-8.

5. Spinner M, Choi BY. Anterior dislocation of the proximal interphalangeal joint. A cause of rupture of the central slip of the extensor mechanism. J Bone Joint Surg Am. 1970;52:1329–36.

6. Elfar J, Mann T. Fracture-dislocations of the proximal interphalangeal joint. J Am Acad Orthop Surg. 2013;21:88–98. doi:10.5435/JAAOS-21-02-88.

7. Green DP. Green's operative hand surgery. 6th ed. Philadelphia, PA: Churchill Livingstone; 2005.

8. Wolfe SW, Dick HM. Articular fractures of the hand. Part I: Guidelines for assessment. Orthop Rev. 1991;20:27–32.

9. Elson RA. Rupture of the central slip of the extensor hood of the finger. A test for early diagnosis. J Bone Joint Surg Br. 1986;68:229–31.

10. Rosenstadt BE, Glickel SZ, Lane LB, Kaplan SJ. Palmar fracture dislocation of the proximal interphalangeal joint. J Hand Surg Am. 1998;23:811–20. doi:10.1016/S0363-5023(98)80155-X.

11. Inoue G, Maeda N. Irreducible palmar dislocation of the proximal interphalangeal joint of the finger. J Hand Surg Am. 1990;15:301–4. doi:10.1016/0363-5023(90)90113-6.

12. Itadera E. Irreducible palmar dislocation of the proximal interphalangeal joint caused by a fracture fragment: a case report. J Orthop Sci. 2003;8:872–4. doi:10.1007/s00776-003-0726-7.

13. Williams 4th CS. Proximal interphalangeal joint fracture dislocations: stable and unstable. Hand Clin. 2012;28:409–16. doi:10.1016/j.hcl.2012.05.036.

14. Birman MV, Rossenwasser MP. Proximal interphalangeal joint fracture dislocations in professional baseball players. Hand Clin. 2012;28:417–20. doi:10.1016/j.hcl.2012.05.037.

15. Khouri JS, Bloom JM, Hammert WC. Current trends in the management of proximal interphalangeal joint injuries of the hand. Plast Reconstr Surg. 2013;132:1192–204. doi:10.1097/PRS.0b013e3182a48d65.

16. Blazar PE, Steinberg DR. Fractures of the proximal interphalangeal joint. J Am Acad Orthop Surg. 2000;8:383–90.

Chapter 16
Operative Treatment of Volar PIP Joint Fracture-Dislocations

Lawrence E. Weiss and Stephanie Sweet

Abstract Volar PIP joint fracture-dislocations are less common than dorsal instability patterns. They usually represent significant injury to the extensor mechanism and are unforgiving unless optimally treated. The operative exposure and technique of dorsal fixation are demonstrated here. An anatomic reduction of the fracture is more likely to result in restoration of the normal length of the extensor mechanism and facilitate healing of the central slip. A short-arc motion protocol can often be initiated if fixation is sound.

Keywords Volar fracture-dislocation • Central slip injury • PIP joint articular fracture • Instability PIP joint

L.E. Weiss, M.D. (✉)
Division of Hand Surgery, OAA Hand Center, Lehigh Valley Hospital,
250 Cetronia Road, Second Floor, Allentown, PA 18104, USA
e-mail: lweiss@oaainstitute.com

S. Sweet, M.D.
Philadelphia Hand Center, Thomas Jefferson University,
700 S. Henderson Road, King of Prussia, PA 19406, USA
e-mail: ssweet@handcenters.com

© Springer International Publishing Switzerland 2016   211
J.E. Adams (ed.), *PIP Joint Fracture Dislocations*,
DOI 10.1007/978-3-319-28579-5_16

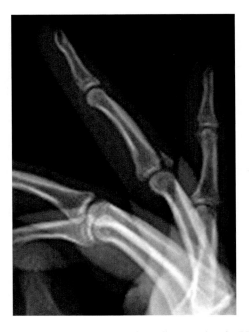

Fig. 16.1 Volar dislocation, with pain and swelling noted at the PIP joint

Case Presentation

This 34-year-old male injured his dominant ring finger playing basketball. He sustained a volar dislocation that was self-reduced. Pain
and swelling were noted at the PIP joint. Range of motion was 15 to
30° actively at the injured joint. Radiographs reveal the following
unstable fracture pattern. Operative treatment was indicated (Fig. 16.1).

Initial Approach

Approach this injury dorsally, separating the central tendon from the
lateral bands. Preserve the attachment of the central slip on the base of
the middle phalanx. The triangular ligament may be split to enable
fracture line delineation to facilitate anatomic reduction (Fig. 16.2).

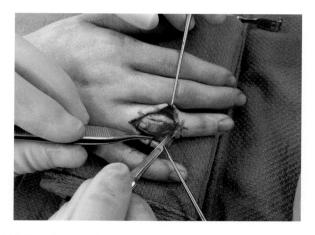

Fig. 16.2 Dorsal approach, separating central tendon from lateral bands

Evaluation of the Dorsal PIP Joint

Once the fracture is delineated, this can be freely elevated to enable evaluation of the PIP joint. This will require capsular incisions to be made superior to the radial and ulnar collateral ligaments to fully elevate the fracture with its attached central slip and joint capsular insertion (Fig. 16.3).

Fracture Reduction

A tenaculum clamp can be used to enable reduction and compression of the fracture. This achieves anatomic joint reduction of the PIP joint. It is permissible to temporarily place the volar tine of the tenaculum clamp percutaneously midline into the volar base of the middle phalanx to facilitate anatomic reduction of the fracture and PIP dislocation (Fig. 16.4).

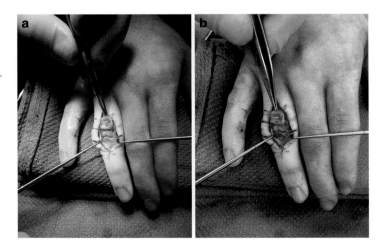

Fig. 16.3 Fracture elevated to enable evaluation of the PIP joint

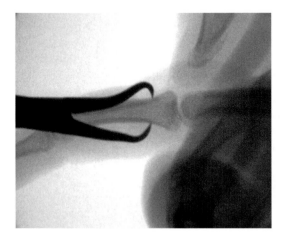

Fig. 16.4 Tenaculum clamp enables reduction and compression of fracture

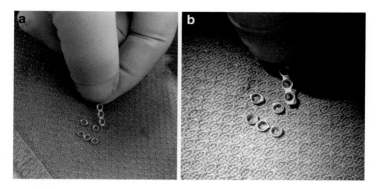

Fig. 16.5 1.3 mm plate is cut into either single- or double-jointed screw eyelets/washers

Choice of Fixation

A 1.3 mm plate is cut into either single- or double-jointed screw eyelets (washers). This can help to enhance fixation support and limit screw cut-through on the dorsal cortex. Lag fixation is achieved with 1.3 mm screws with or without washers (Fig. 16.5).

Fracture Fixation

Fixation is then achieved with as many fixation points as the fragment size allows. The use of washers is selected as required based on the local thickness of the dorsal cortex (Fig. 16.6).

Extensor Repair

The lateral bands and triangular ligament are repaired to the adjacent sides of the central slip. Placement of the DIP joint in flexion enables proper tensioning of the intrinsic component of the extensor mechanism to suture the lateral bands in place (Fig. 16.7).

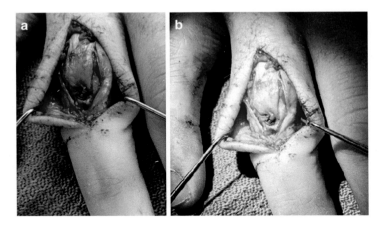

Fig. 16.6 Fixation employing as many fixation points as the fragment size allows. Use washers required based on local thickness of the dorsal cortex

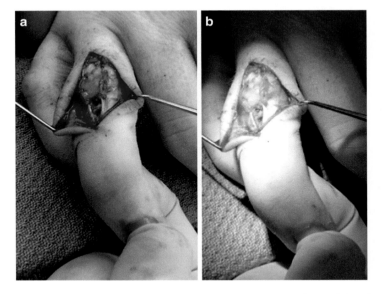

Fig. 16.7 Lateral bands and triangular ligament repaired to adjacent sides of the central slip

Checking the Extensor Balance

The extensor balance should be checked after securing the lateral bands. Bring the PIP joint into flexion and confirm that lateral band excursion is satisfactory by checking tension at the DIP joint. This also confirms satisfactory restoration of central slip support at the base of the middle phalanx (Fig. 16.8).

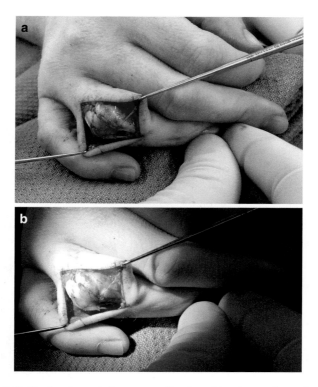

Fig. 16.8 Check extensor balance to confirm lateral band excursion and restoration of central slip support

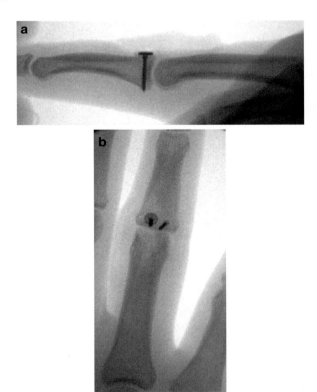

Fig. 16.9 Final alignment after procedure

Final Alignment (Fig. 16.9)

Postoperative Care

Soft dressings and a supportive finger splint are applied at surgery. The patient may be seen in hand therapy within a few days postoperatively to begin a progressive short-arc range of motion recovery program for the PIP joint. Emphasis on lateral band mobilization includes digital abduction-adduction as well as DIP mobilization. Goals of therapy are full range of motion within 6 weeks and firm grasp restoration by 3 months.

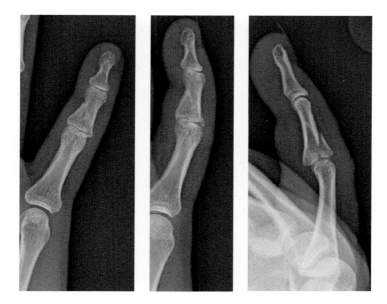

Fig. 16.10 Fifth finger volar PIP fracture-dislocation

Case Presentation #2

A 26-year-old female sustained a fifth finger volar PIP fracture-dislocation during dodge-ball. The middle phalanx base fracture configuration had an oblique metaphyseal component (Fig. 16.10).

Fixation with lag screw fixation through the base component along with lag fixation of the dorsal avulsion component was completed, according to the technique previously outlined. Postoperative care was initiated as described previously (Fig. 16.11).

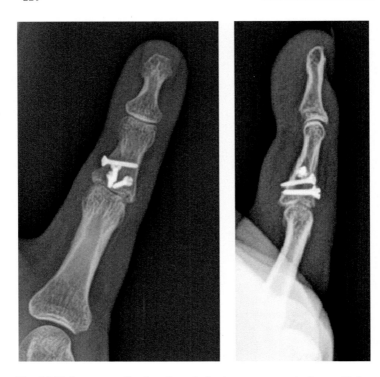

Fig. 16.11 Lag screw fixation through the base component along with lag fixation of the dorsal avulsion component

Suggested Readings

1. Grant I, Berger AC, Tham SK. Internal fixation of unstable fracture dislocations of the proximal interphalangeal joint. J Hand Surg Br. 2005;30B:492–8.
2. Rosenstadt BE, Glickel SZ, Lane LB, Kaplan SJ. Palmar fracture dislocation of the proximal interphalangeal joint. J Hand Surg Am. 1998;23A:811–20.
3. Hastings H, Carroll C. Treatment of closed articular fractures of the metacarpophalangeal and proximal interphalangeal joints. Hand Clin. 1988;4:503–27.

4. Kiefhaber TR, Stern PJ. Fracture dislocations of the proximal interpha-langeal joint. J Hand Surg Am. 1988;23A:368–80.
5. Calfee RP, Sommerkamp TG. Fracture-dislocation about the finger joints. J Hand Surg Am. 2009;34A:1140–7.
6. Tekkis PP, Kessaris N, Gavalas M, et al. The role of mini-fragment screw fixation in volar dislocations of the proximal interphalangeal joint. Arch Orthop Trauma Surg. 2001;121:121–2.

Index

© Springer International Publishing Switzerland 2016
J.E. Adams (ed.), *PIP Joint Fracture Dislocations*,
DOI 10.1007/978-3-319-28579-5

Printed in the United States
By Bookmasters